THE ON-SITE PHYSICAL THERAPIST

Dr. Christine McCallum PT, DPT

THE ON-SITE PHYSICAL THERAPIST

DIRECT-TO-EMPLOYER CARE

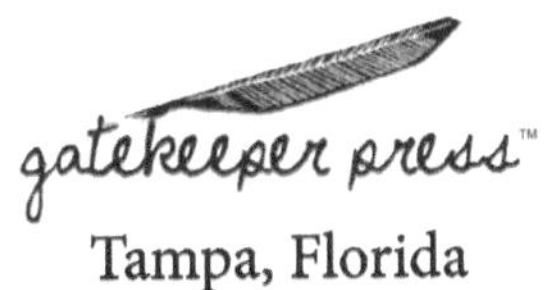

Tampa, Florida

THE ON-SITE PHYSICAL THERAPIST:
Direct-To-Employer Care

Published by Gatekeeper Press
7853 Gunn Hwy, Suite 209
Tampa, FL 33626
www.GatekeeperPress.com

Library of Congress Control Number: 2023940347

ISBN (paperback): 9798218182656
eISBN: 9798218182663

This book is dedicated to all my patients who inspire me to be better; I send a sincere thank you to my family and friends for their support and encouragement throughout my career and this book writing process. And, deep gratitude to my Book Coach, Beth Brand. This project would not have come to fruition without her expertise and gentle nudging.

CONTENTS

The On-Site Physical Therapist

*Get out of the clinic and into a practice model
where you are essential to the crew, get paid your worth,
and love your work again.*

....

—Christine McCallum, PT, DPT

INTRODUCTION

Sadly, physical therapists have been pushed into double-booked, overstressed practitioners who have to compromise the best possible care for so much less. To really do good work, you must have time to work with patients one-on-one. This on-site model of practice allows the PT to work at a higher level of skill on behalf of the patient.

—Richelle Sipiora, PT (my mentor and longtime friend)

When I was in eighth grade, I told my mom I wanted to be a PE teacher. She countered with, "What about a physical therapist?" I asked her what that was. She said, "People who help people like your aunt Rita."

My aunt Rita had severe cerebral palsy. I always enjoyed pushing her wheelchair, helping her walk, holding the leash while rolling-walking her dog, and listening to her tell a joke—she was slow to speak but oh so witty. From the moment my mom suggested physical therapy (PT), I knew it was right for me. I felt it was my calling.

I went through the required undergraduate work and applied to PT school. I earned a master's in physical therapy. And as the adage goes (or as Aristotle said), "The more you know, the more you realize you don't know." This was certainly true for me. That's why after several years in practice, I went back to school to get my doctorate. Like most of us who are called to this field, I'm a lifelong learner. In PT, there are always new findings, new skills to master, and better treatment protocols to discover.

My PT career began in hospitals, where I gained experience in inpatient care, acute rehab, post-operation orthopedics, intensive care, and oncology care. I then transferred to brick-and-mortar outpatient clinics, where my focus was occupational health, workers' compensation, and orthopedic PT. Along the way, I was lucky to work with talented teammates who willingly shared their knowledge and industry insights with me.

About a decade into my career, I—like so many of my colleagues, maybe like you—found myself burned out, stressed out, disheartened with the profession, and ready to call it quits. If you work in PT, then you know the constraints put on our practice by insurance companies and other financial concerns. You've experienced the pressure of seeing too many patients in a day and the never-ending paperwork. You've had to cope with the relatively low pay for professionals with our level of education and skill, coupled with too many hours. And you've seen these issues drive many talented PTs from the profession.

At the ten-year mark, I felt more like a generic cog in the medical industry merry-go-round than a valued professional. Between the insurance mandates and time limitations, I couldn't give my patients the level of care I knew was possible. I finally got to where I couldn't see myself working under these conditions one more day, let alone the rest of my life. So I considered giving up my PT career, despite how much I loved caring for patients.

ON-SITE PT

Luckily, I didn't have to quit PT. As I was looking for another line of work, I found an area of practice I hadn't known about—a way of practicing that demands and allows me to use the full extent of my knowledge and skill. While I still treat patients for injuries, the focus and success of my work now is measured by my ability to prevent injuries and increase patient wellness overall. Maybe most remarkable, I'm paid my worth and have control over my hours. The area of practice I found—fell into, really—was on-site physical therapy.

On-site physical therapists practice in clinics located inside major production facilities, warehouses, and distribution centers. It is "direct-to-employer" care. Our clients are typically corporations that self-insure—which allows freedom to provide services creatively, outside of the typical insurance-care algorithms. Our patients are the corporation's workers. Our mandate is to keep their employees healthy and injury free. As an on-site PT, I did have to give up being an employee and become an independent contractor—meaning I run my own small business. At first, this scared me. But today, I tout it as one of the greatest benefits to my career and life.

Though on-site care has been around for decades and all trends point to its continued growth, on-site practice just isn't well-known among physical therapists. Most companies do not use on-site PT clinics, and most insurance claim managers do not suggest on-site PT clinics as a way to decrease costs. PT students don't learn about it in school. Most books I've found on building a PT practice focus on cash pay, concierge, or mobile PT.

I wrote *The On-Site Physical Therapist* to let my fellow PTs—especially those who are feeling burned out in more traditional areas of practice—know that on-site, direct-to-employer care exists, as well as how it can change their lives and careers for the better. So many of the negative factors that make PTs leave the profession aren't part of on-site practice. In contrast, so much of why we become PTs in the first place is integral to providing great on-site care.

In this book, you'll learn what on-site PT is, how it works, and where the opportunities are in the field today. If what you read about this type of practice resonates with you, you'll also find within this book a practical, step-by-step guide to opening your own on-site practice. You'll learn both what it takes and what you need to get started.

EVERYTHING YOU NEED TO KNOW

The book is divided into three sections:

Section 1: "The Opportunity" defines on-site PT. It then takes you on a deep dive into how the field came to be and how it's practiced today. You get a thorough understanding of why companies choose to both self-insure and offer health care on location—as well as what that means for you, the on-site practitioner.

Section 2: "The On-Site PT Business Model" leads you through all the various components involved in an on-site PT practice. You learn what's expected of an on-site PT through an in-depth look at who your clients and patients are. A general overview of the state and federal agencies and laws that govern on-site care makes you aware of the scope of your on-site practice. You also come to understand and learn to calculate the value of your services in dollars and cents. Finally, you see the various ways you can structure a practice—along with the pros and cons of each setup.

Section 3: "Operating Your On-Site Business" is about the nuts and bolts of actually opening your practice. The first chapter in this section reviews the professionals you need on your team—where to find them, what to ask them, and how to use them. In subsequent chapters, you get an equipment checklist for setting up your home office and your on-site clinic. You see where your clients will come from, how to choose the ideal clients for you, and how to approach them. You learn what goes into and how to write a winning proposal and a solid contract. And you get insight and some dos and don'ts for your first day on the job and at your clinic.

Every chapter in every section uses examples from my own experiences building an on-site practice. My mistakes and achievements, along with real client and patient interactions, help you avoid the common pitfalls I fell into and take full advantage of those places where I did get it right. Of course, names and details of any client or patient interactions have been changed to protect their privacy. Each chapter ends with an exercise—both questions to help you use the information to achieve your personal goals and activities to help you build the foundation of a plan for your own on-site practice.

MANIFEST YOUR ON-SITE CAREER

Early in my on-site career, I was an employee who worked for a wellness company and provided on-site PT. Today, I run my own small business. I have contracts with multiple clients, as well as a few subcontracts. I also have several employees who I train to staff at each client location (all of which you'll learn more about). My point here is as on-site PT, you can build the career and business you want on your terms. You can grow and add contracts and employees. Or you can choose to be a business of one. With on-site, you define success for you. Whatever you decide, you're in charge of your career, your income, and your hours, which means you're in charge of your life. Being an independent contractor and running a small business isn't for everyone. However, those of us who find ourselves drawn to on-site PT find a career that's more dynamic and opportunity-filled than any other area of physical therapy practice.

I'm at twenty years and counting now as an on-site PT. I've never looked back, and I've loved every minute of it. The requirements and opportunities of on-site care have changed the way I both perceive and practice PT. Being able to see patients immediately when they need my care—coupled with the duty to make their workplace as safe as possible in the first place—lets me feel my skills matter every day.

I'm still as challenged by the work as I am excited and proud to be doing it. On-site has kept me growing as a PT professional and as a person. All signs point to it continuing to do so. That's why I want to educate as many PTs as possible about on-site PT services and give them the information necessary to start their own on-site practice.

So turn the page. Find out what on-site PT is and is all about. You, too, may find your calling here. I hope you do.

Section One

THE OPPORTUNITY

As physical therapists (PTs), we leave school with a range of options for practice: hospital care, rehabilitation, home health, nursing-care facilities, and (where most of us land) the brick-and-mortar outpatient clinic. One option that doesn't often appear on that standard list is the on-site practice: a PT clinic inside a company that serves the company's employees.

I'm not sure why on-site, direct-to-employer care isn't better promoted. Maybe because it asks more of us as professionals. With on-site, direct-to-employer care, the PT is in charge. Our responsibilities to our patients and their companies go far beyond treating injuries. We're asked to (and get to) take on challenges and solve problems that would never cross our path in any other area of practice.

While that may not be attractive to everyone, those things are also the very reasons many PTs choose to provide direct-to-employer care via an on-site PT clinic. It asks more of us because it delivers more to us—more ways to use our knowledge and skill, more possibilities for affecting the well-being of our patients and improving their working environment, and more compensation.

With so many choices, every PT can and should find the type of practice that suits them best. This first section gives you the basics of the on-site PT clinic—defining the job and the scope of opportunities the on-site practice offers.

1

WHY ON-SITE PT

A little more than two decades ago, I woke up with hands so stiff I could barely pick up my coffee mug. This didn't surprise me completely. I hadn't been able to play my guitar in months due to the pain. As I carefully lifted my cup to my mouth—using two hands—I thought, "Here I am, a practicing physical therapist who can't hold a mug of coffee." That was strike one.

Later that morning at work, I was reviewing my patient notes in preparation for my appointments that day. From the notes, I couldn't tell which returning patient was which. As usual and in every case, I'd been in a rush to finish my notes because there was always another patient waiting. Thus, the notes contained more rote documentation than clinical information. I hadn't had time to record specific observations on patient status, movement dysfunction, or care needed. Looking at the notes now, I realized I'd have to wait until I put my hands on each patient and watch them move to know which direction to go with their treatment. Strike two.

A few days after that, I became ill at work. I needed to go home. Now, I can count on one hand how many sick days I've had in my career. I was feeling awful. When I let my supervisor know, their first—and exact—

words were, "You didn't cancel your patients for the day, did you? We need to keep them on the schedule."

My supervisor didn't ask what was wrong or express concern for me. This trained health care provider did not ask if I needed treatment or help. No, the focus was on making sure my condition did not affect the clinic's bottom line.

Standing there with chills and a raging headache, listening to those words come out of my supervisor's mouth, I could no longer deny that this clinic's primary focus was revenue. If I was going to grow professionally and rise through the ranks here, I'd need to become impervious to the pressures and adopt the high-volume patient care mindset and billing practices as well.

For me, that was it. Strike three.

At this point, I'd been licensed and working in PT clinics for a decade. The only thing I'd ever wanted to be was a physical therapist. I loved the work itself, the patient interaction, and using my knowledge and skill to restore a person to full function and relieve their pain. But now this job I loved so much was causing me pain. The high overhead and top-heavy bureaucracy of the brick-and-mortar PT clinic was limiting quality time with patients, not allowing me to do my best work, treating me like a commodity, all while robbing my hands of mobility and my life of joy.

IS THIS JUST THE WAY IT IS?

I, of course, was not the first PT to face this truth about how we're expected to practice. Many PTs before me, and maybe even you, have arrived at strike three—or at least, strike two—with the rigid, insurance-dependent clinic model.

It's no wonder. We're highly educated professionals with much to offer our patients. Yet more often than not, we're constrained on multiple fronts from using our full knowledge and talents. Our schedules and appointments are at the mercy of the clinic's insurance contracts and the size of the bureaucracy the clinic supports. The scope of care we're able to offer is driven not by individual patient need alone, but by the number of patients we're asked to see in a day. I've given instructions for many home exercise programs while cleaning the treatment table or walking backward to get my next patient in the waiting room—and I'm sure you have too.

We're paid a salary for forty hours a week. Yet for most of us, it takes forty-five to fifty hours each week to do the job completely and professionally. PTs often complete patient notes and plan of care documents at home, off the clock—after doing the laundry, cleaning up after dinner, or putting the kids to bed. Ironically, this high volume and fast pace also puts PTs at high risk for work-related injuries, my own hands being a case in point.

Like most health care entities in the United States, a typical outpatient PT clinic depends on insurance contracts, Medicare reimbursement rates, or the patient paying cash out of pocket. To remain financially viable, clinics are set up to maximize the number of patients coming in the door for care. Because of that, the PT's primary focus (and all the appointment length allows for) is to treat people after an injury has occurred, with the goal of improving function, managing pain, and, when possible, increasing the patient's self-care ability. Little to no time is allotted for considering the patient's lifestyle, deriving the root cause of the injury, or better yet, preventing the injury in the first place.

Experience has shown me that even those brick-and-mortar clinics that strive to provide better employee reimbursement and shield providers from overhead costs/bureaucracy driving every decision eventually yield to market forces. No matter how brightly a brick-and-mortar clinic presents itself, eventually things regress—contracts, corporate costs, and budgets change; new leadership comes in; and the clinic's reimbursement and bureaucratic procedures tighten. Then, the pressure to see more patients in less time returns—along with a drop in job satisfaction and a rise in both physical and mental stress on the PTs and other clinic employees. Once a colleague of mine overheard a corporate executive say while touring her clinic, "If people are going to get better, we might as well have a PT clinic and charge them for it." That type of corporate philosophy was breaking me to the point of no return.

Of course, not every brick-and-mortar PT clinic is that disheartening to work for. The vast majority are just trying to make it in a business model where the only way to increase revenue is to increase patient load. For some PTs, working in a traditional clinic is a good fit. For many of us, however (including me), it is not.

What I was looking for—and what I'm guessing you may be looking for too—is a model of practice where patients are seen and treated in their entirety, not just as an injury; where PTs are valued as trusted professionals; where we can spend time with our patients and not be rushed. Where PTs make treatment decisions based on what they determine to be best for those in their care, not on what an insurance representative approves. A practice where preventing injury and healing patients is more valuable to the clinic's business model than moving through an impossibly high patient volume each day. As long as I was dreaming, I also wanted to have some control over my work schedule and be compensated well.

I didn't realize it at the time, but what I was describing was an on-site physical therapy practice.

INSIDE ON-SITE

As the name suggests, on-site physical therapists practice on-site, where our patients work—which is typically a manufacturing facility, factory, or warehouse, wherever job completion is dependent on physical labor. While the brick-and-mortar PT clinic model makes money via contracted rates through treating injuries after the fact, the on-site model measures success by saving costs through preventing injury wherever possible and providing immediate treatment when injury does occur.

On-site PT clinics come in all shapes and sizes. Some exist in conjunction with larger on-site medical clinics or fitness facilities. Some consist of one therapist in a small space on or near the production or work area. Most employers who offer on-site care are self-insured—meaning they fund their own employee and workers' compensation medical plans (more on this in Chapter 4). Consequently, on-site PT care is not paid for, determined by, or limited by insurance companies—which means "care" can take on a more diverse and satisfying meaning.

Employees can and do come to the on-site PT clinic for work-related injuries. They also use our services to relieve whatever pain they're experiencing. And they receive this care at no charge or for a small fee. Whatever the reason for the appointment, our mandate as on-site PTs is to keep the workforce healthy and working. We're given the time and resources to provide the care necessary to see it through. To me and most physical therapists I know, the on-site model allows us to practice the way we envisioned when we were in PT school.

On-site PTs are not direct employees of the company or facility where we have our on-site clinic. We are either self-employed, independent contractors who contract directly with the corporation (our client), or we are employees of a wellness company or medical provider that places us on-site. This arrangement limits liability for the corporation (the client). It also supports autonomy in our decision-making. As a bonus, our patients see us as independent from their employer, bolstering their trust in us.

Though not employed by the corporation, as an on-site PT, you do ultimately become a member of the workforce you serve. You work side by side with the people you're charged with caring for. You come to know the demands of their jobs, how they move throughout their day, and the expectations put on them for productivity. You also come to know them as people—you learn about their families, their lifestyles, their personal challenges. This inside knowledge adds exponentially to your effectiveness in caring for them.

Most gratifying of all is that because the employees (your patients) feel comfortable around you, when they need your services, they're more likely to come for intervention before an injury becomes a crisis. Studies have shown that just having an on-site PT clinic makes employees more likely to participate in other company health benefit plans and programs in general, improving their health beyond PT services.

THE RISE OF THE ON-SITE PT

Though not well known, physical therapy at the worksite isn't that new. It was introduced into the military nearly half a century ago and took root in the manufacturing world several decades ago. As David G. Greathouse and Brian Young explained in their essay published in the March 2021 issues of *PTJ (Physical Therapy & Rehabilitation Journal)*, during the Vietnam War, the military found itself with a shortage of physicians and orthopedic specialists. At the same time, PT expertise was advancing by leaps and bounds. So the military decided to use PTs in a direct-access capacity—meaning no doctor's prescription needed for treatment. PTs would be the first point of contact for musculoskeletal (MSK) conditions, which were plentiful due to injuries related to physical fitness training, as well as the physical injuries of service.

When that limited program proved successful, PTs became involved with all active troops. Right from the start, the military found direct access to PTs decreased delays not only for care of MSK injuries, but also for primary care and referral for treatment. In time, PTs became regular members of military units—training with them, making recommendations for fitness programs, and implementing injury prevention and care programs. According to Greathouse and Young, studies showed that direct access to PTs in the military decreased the need for air evacuation to higher levels of care, diagnostic imaging, and prescription medications. Units with PTs embedded enjoyed better return-to-duty rates for MSK injuries than those without PTs. Today, PTs are deployed on foreign bases and on all types of missions, from humanitarian to combat, and are part of special operations units in all branches of the military.

As soon as it was clear that direct access was a triumph for the military, the American Physical Therapy Association (APTA) began lobbying to gain direct access to physical therapy for the general population in the United States—and it was successful. As of this writing, all states and territories allow some form of direct access to evaluation by a PT. However, when it comes to specific treatments, ordering images, and prescribing medications for MSK disorders, each state and territory has its own laws.

Direct access is what makes it possible for businesses to have on-site PT clinics. However, over the last few decades, it's the rising cost of private health insurance that's driven the on-site movement in the private sector. As insurance rates rise and benefits decline, more companies are finding it financially advantageous to self-insure. (We'll talk more about direct-access laws, the inner working of self-insurance, and what the on-site PT needs to know about both in upcoming chapters.)

As you might imagine, when a corporation foots its own health care bill, prevention takes on a whole new urgency, so investing in on-site care makes sense. Over the years, study after study has shown that—just like in the military—on-site care within corporations decreases the number of claims overall. These clinics keep workers on the job, which keeps production high and corporate profits up. As these benefits become better known, the demand for on-site PT clinics rises, and so do the opportunities for physical therapists.

As further evidence of the PT profession's growing influence in and importance to workplace health care, in February 2023, the American Physical Therapy Association (APTA) became an affiliate of the Centers for Disease Control's Total Worker Health Initiative, along with other major health care organizations and academic institutions. The APTA's participation in this initiative positions the organization to even more effectively advocate for PTs as primary care and entry point providers—especially in the area of on-site care.

MAKING THE LEAP TO AN ON-SITE CAREER

Like most of my colleagues, I had no idea that on-site PT was an option for me until I fell into it. My job-hunting attempts at first were chaotic, to say the least. Uninspired by the conditions I found at other brick-and-mortar clinics, I looked into weight training as a PT. I also took a vocational rehab course, where I learned my ideal job would be as a river guide. While I was sure that being a river guide would be personally fulfilling and a ton of fun, I wasn't so sure how well it would cover my mortgage.

Then, several weeks into my search, I came across an ad: "Wanted: experienced physical therapist, in corporate wellness setting, ergonomic experience a plus." I applied, not sure of what I was getting into but more than ready to get out of where I was. At the interview, I learned the ad was from a corporate wellness company that placed on-site physical therapists. After an extended process, I got the job.

My first assignment was in a bare-bones start-up clinic on the floor of a major beverage producer. I'd spend the next ten years in that location, working closely with the company's employees, who were responsible for producing packaging, shipping, and distributing products. In that time, I was given the opportunity to grow the corporation's on-site PT program from the ground up. I learned about job coaching, pre-employment testing, functional capacity evaluations, and work conditioning—opportunities I would not have had at a brick-and-mortar clinic. I also, of course, treated a wide variety of work-related and non-work-related injuries.

Most importantly, I found a job and an environment where I was professionally fulfilled. I had the time and space to use all my skills and professional judgment not only to heal my patient's injuries and alleviate their pain, but to work with those patients to ensure their injuries didn't reoccur. I was regularly consulted and listened to by managers regarding how to prevent employee injury as they designed workflow and set production goals. Every day, I was a contributing member of a team, valued for the knowledge I brought to the table. This is typical of the on-site experience.

When I started my on-site career, I was an employee of a wellness company. As their employee, I went where they assigned me and was paid a salary they set. It was a fair salary. I worked eight hours each day, more or less. Twice a month, I received a paycheck. While you can still find opportunities to be "employed" as an on-site PT (my own company currently hires

PTs as employees), there's more to be gained by being a self-employed, independent contractor in this field. You'll see that's the career path I encourage throughout this book.

I made the switch to independent contractor around 2014, when being an employee ceased to be an option because the law in Colorado (where I live and work) changed. That law stated that a business could not operate a PT clinic unless the owner was a licensed physical therapist. The owners of the wellness company I worked for were not. So, if I wanted to continue to serve the client on-site, I'd have to become my own business and an independent contractor to the wellness company.

Like most physical therapists, I'd only ever worked for someone else. The idea of being responsible for my own business and my entire income left me scared. We don't get much business education in PT school. I'd never even been laid off or lost my job. My only experience running a small business was a side hustle I'd tried years before—the "Musician Mender." I gave massages to local musicians to get them to consider physical therapy to help with their performance-related MSK issues. The problem was few musicians had the money for even an inexpensive massage, and even fewer had health insurance for regular PT. Despite the clever business name, my only attempt at entrepreneurship had been a dud.

To say I was apprehensive about making such a move would be an understatement—so I get how this one aspect of becoming an on-site PT might be concerning to you right now. At that time, I wished with all my heart that things could remain status quo. Then, just when I needed it, the client liaison at the on-site clinic told me how much she valued my work and that the PT clinic I'd developed had become an anchor in their business. She wanted me to stay. My supervisors at the wellness company also praised my work and encouraged me to make the change to independent contractor. With their support—and no other choice—I took the leap.

So let me reassure you here and now. You can do this. Yes, it felt like an immense leap. But it was a leap I would make again a thousand times over and one I have recommended to countless other PTs wanting more from their career. With that one decision, I was able to improve my pay, provide more comprehensive care for my patients, and be the autonomous provider I'd always wanted to be. Over the years, my business has grown and so have I, both professionally and personally. In addition to contracting through a wellness company when the subcontract suits my business, I now also contract directly with multiple corporations with on-site clinics (my clients), where I place myself and my employees.

If becoming an independent contractor right away still feels overwhelming, you can look for a wellness/therapy company in your area to hire you as an employee. It's a good way to test the waters of on-site practice and see what this kind of practice is all about. However, only as an independent contractor will you receive the full benefit of what an on-site PT practice offers—the opportunity to take charge of your work, your income, and your life.

I promise it's not as scary or difficult as it might seem from where you are now. The physical therapy part you already know. The business part can be learned easily enough—as you'll discover in upcoming chapters. Most PTs who've become independent, on-site PTs (including me) see it as the best career move they've ever made—a huge professional advance. I'm here to support you all the way.

....

EXERCISE
Is On-Site PT for Me?

....

At the end of each chapter is an exercise for you: a series of questions and activities. (You'll notice more "questions" in this first section and more "activities" as we move through the book and build your on-site PT practice.) I encourage you to write out your answers to the questions and do the activities. Taken all together as you finish the book, your work will provide the direction you need as you make decisions about whether to become an on-site PT and what steps you need to build an on-site PT practice.

Questions

1. Why did you become a PT?
2. What do you love most about your current PT position?
3. What do you find frustrating? What would you change?
4. Have you considered leaving the field? Why?
5. What makes you stay?
6. Describe your perfect PT job.
7. From what you read in Chapter 1, what about on-site PT intrigues you? What gives you the most concern?
8. How do you feel about being a business owner?
9. Does the idea of becoming an on-site PT excite you? Why or why not?

Activity

- Do some research and identify a few on-site PT clinics in your area.

2

———

THE JOB

One afternoon, an employee stopped by the on-site PT clinic to see if I could help him with some rib pain he was experiencing. He told me he'd first noticed it when he woke up that morning. Now, several hours into his shift, the pain was making it a little hard to breathe. He explained he wouldn't have bothered with it, but he was going on vacation the next day and didn't want to take this pain with him.

The patient interview uncovered some other issues he'd been experiencing over the last several weeks—such as headaches, decreased balance, and difficulty stopping when walking downhill. He said he'd been "meaning to see his doctor" but "hadn't gotten around to making an appointment." When I pressed for more details, he let me know that nine weeks earlier, he'd fallen while skiing. He'd been wearing a helmet at the time but still suffered a mild concussion. He did see his doctor after that injury. The concussion symptoms had lasted about two weeks. He said he was fine now.

Alerted and concerned by what his history revealed, I decided to conduct a thorough neuro evaluation. Then I called his physician with my findings. An MRI was arranged for that night. It showed a bilateral intracra-

23

nial hemorrhage. So, instead of getting on a plane for a nine-hour flight the next day, the employee had surgery to relieve pressure on his brain.

BETTER CARE FOR PATIENTS

I don't know if the on-site PT clinic model saved that employee's life that day, but I do know that it put him in the best situation possible. My patient had direct, easy access to my services on the same day he needed them. No referral or authorization was necessary that would delay his health care needs. He didn't worry about cost because he knew the care would be affordable for him. He was seen by a provider (me) who was familiar with him. I'd observed him daily on the shop floor and at the on-site gym. So I knew by looking at him that afternoon that there was more wrong than a painful rib or a pulled muscle. In that same vein, I wasn't constrained by scheduling issues. I wasn't just checking off boxes during the patient interview. I had the freedom to take my time and listen to him. I had the freedom to dig as deep as was needed to determine an appropriate differential diagnosis. I also had complete autonomy to decide next steps—including calling the patient's physician to order imaging.

As PTs, we all know how we'd like to practice—being accessible to our patients; having the time needed to ensure proper clinical diagnosis, treatment, and follow up; being part of an integrated system that allows cross-referral and collaboration; and having the ability to use our full professional knowledge to educate and empower our patients to take care of themselves and prevent injury in the first place. The on-site clinic practice is structured to make room for exactly that level of patient care. That's the job.

Much of the on-site practice structure can be credited to the fact that the clinic's revenue source (the self-insured company) and the health care provider are not working at cross purposes. The mission—how everyone profits—is maintaining a workforce that's fit to work. Our sole goal is to do everything within our abilities to increase patient wellness. Patient health is our first consideration in all decisions—with the rest of the operation flowing from there.

AN EXPANDED SCOPE OF PRACTICE

On-site PTs do treat patients in our clinics who make appointments, of course. But we don't sit in our clinics all day waiting for patients to show up. We are out on the floor, among the employees, in their workspaces, watching people move. We are skilled observers, actively looking for opportunities to improve employee performance, relieve pain, and prevent injury. As we make our rounds, we find countless openings to bring our skills to situations and people—many who didn't know they needed us.

Once when I was out in the production area, I observed an employee limping at the end of his workday. I'd done his pre-employment test, so I knew this wasn't normal for him. When I asked what was going on, he said, "Oh, my feet are bad, just like everyone in my family. There's nothing I can do. I'll probably need surgery eventually." I asked him to come by the clinic as soon as he could.

He came in before his shift the next morning. Upon examination, I concluded that "bad feet" was an understatement. With fallen arches, bunions, neuropathy, and callus development, his situation was difficult—and yet, he'd never sought treatment for any of these very painful and debilitating issues. Like everyone else in his family, he simply accepted the pain and figured one day it would get to the point where he'd "need surgery."

Right away, I performed some manual PT and provided some exercises to unload his forefoot. I then educated him as to what footwear and supportive shoe inserts would improve his comfort and walking. I showed him how to manage his calluses.

He left my clinic and returned to work that day with significantly less pain and in a much better mood. In a few days, upon securing the shoes and the inserts and employing the prescribed exercises and care routine, he reported that his pain had decreased significantly. He said he felt so much better and had more energy. He hadn't realized how the foot pain had been limiting his activities by keeping him from taking any extra steps at work and home.

The PT intervention took about two hours over the course of three weeks. I was able to give him the care he needed without causing him to lose days of work running to outside doctor's appointments. I'd also argue the care made him more productive on the job—more than making up for the cost of those two hours. As for me, I got the satisfaction of helping a patient who didn't know his pain could be taken care of with nothing more invasive than a little PT, some orthotics, and some exercises.

Our nature as PTs is to want to help everyone with their discomfort and movement issues. Heaven knows we PTs analyze the movement of every person we encounter—we can't stop ourselves. And while we'd like nothing more than to help those we flag as needing some physical therapy, most of us have enough self-restraint to not approach a perfect stranger in the grocery store and ask about their limp.

In most types of PT practices, we don't get to use our skills unless someone seeks them out. But the on-site practice makes our natural inclination to want to step in part of the job. That employee was lucky to work for a company that valued his well-being enough to hire an on-site PT and make it my business to ask about his limp.

It's also our business to identify "accidents waiting to happen," and apply industry standards and creative strategies to eliminate them. For instance, during a pre-employment physical abilities test, a candidate for a warehouse job struggled to lift a fifty-pound test crate and place it on a shelf. Obviously, he did not safely meet the maximum-lift requirement for the job's critical demands. He was an accident waiting to happen.

I stopped the test and talked to him about his difficulty. He agreed that lifting the crate was "really hard" and doing that repeatedly throughout the day would prove even harder, maybe even dangerous. We agreed the warehouse job wasn't a good fit for him. So I went with him to talk with the supervisor who'd interviewed him to explain the situation. Not wanting to lose an otherwise terrific candidate, the supervisor found another position in the warehouse more suited to the candidate's physical abilities.

Now two years on the job, the employee has become a prized team member and has had no lost time due to injury. That's a huge value to the company, to the employee, and to his supervisor. It's also endlessly gratifying for me. It's a different way of using my PT skills to make a difference in people's lives.

PROBLEM-SEEKING, PROBLEM-SOLVING

As we make our daily rounds, we're also keeping an eye out for ergonomic problems at workstations and devising and implementing solutions to keep employees safe and improve the environment for everyone.

When an employee came to me with wrist pain, I suspected an ergonomic risk related to repetitive or forceful upper extremity use. After a brief session of first aid in the clinic, I headed out to the floor to inspect my patient's actual workstation—as only an on-site PT can do. I noticed that he and his colleagues were working with an eight-inch circumference cylinder, turning it ninety degrees with one hand, and then drilling a small hole into it. Maybe my patient was the only one feeling pain at the moment, but I could see that this method of object handling had the potential to put stress on everyone's wrists.

I suggested putting a small rim on the workstation, like a backstop, to keep the item stable and decrease the grip force by 30 percent (yes, you can measure this.) This not only improved my patient's forearm comfort, rid him of wrist pain, and decreased the ergonomic risk score; it also prevented everyone else in the department from potentially having the same injury and discomfort.

In a more disturbing scenario, a department experienced seven electric pallet jack (EPJ) accidents in three months. Two of them resulted in severe injuries requiring extensive surgery. (EPJ accidents have caused amputation, internal injury, and, on rare occasions, death.) Because of that series of accidents, I began to pay special attention to that department whenever I was nearby. What I observed was unsafe behavior by both new hires and veteran workers.

Upon further research, I found that the EPJ trainees were given very little time during their training to practice driving. Additionally, I found the trainer did not reinforce to anyone on the crew the severity of injury that can occur from making a mistake when operating an EPJ. The trainer's casual style was undermining the company's message of safety first.

Without naming names, I wrote up my observations in a report to the production safety manager. I recommended developing stricter guidelines for the training program and stricter enforcement of behaviors using EPJs. They agreed. Since the new training program has been operational, no more EPJ injuries have occurred in that department.

As you can imagine, this problem-seeking and problem-solving part of the job keeps on-site PTs growing in new and interesting ways as a physical therapist. It's also consequential to our clients and patients in very real ways, running the gamut from saving downtime on a production line to saving lives. I've always said that if people took better care of themselves, I'd gladly change my profession. I don't think accidents and injuries are going to stop happening anytime soon—on the job or at home. However, as on-site PTs, we do get to help humankind inch a little closer to that goal.

BETTER CARE FOR PTs

While the on-site clinic model provides a high level of care for both patients and clients, the model ensures the PT is cared for as well. We are seen by the company we contract with as an investment, not an expense. That standing is reflected in how we are both treated and compensated.

Because what we do is valued, on-site PTs are given the time, the space, and the equipment to do our jobs. High-volume, superficial care has no place in on-site treatment. While our specific hours are built around our client's shift needs, we control our workflow. Yes, some days are busier than others, but we are in charge. There is no pressure to rush through an appointment or cut corners.

The on-site structure also ensures PTs are more reliably and sustainably compensated. Our pay is not determined by how many patients we see and their contracted insurance rates but by the value we add to our client's business and how we negotiate for that value. The more value we can show—the more profit we help them generate by keeping their workforce healthy and their production lines running—the more compensation we can command. (You'll learn how to calculate your value in Chapter 6.)

In the decade since I switched to on-site, my own profit margin has averaged 25 to 30 percent higher than typical brick-and-mortar profit margins. By the way, not being tied to outside insurance eliminates hours of paperwork as well. Not to mention, any paperwork I am responsible for is figured into my fee.

Inside the clinic and the company, the job provides an environment where there is more respect for PTs, which makes on-site practice professionally satisfying. Outside the clinic, the job's more manageable schedule and higher compensation relieve a host of personal stressors and improve our lives.

THE ON-SITE MODEL ISN'T PERFECT

For all its benefits and opportunities, there are some downsides to on-site practice to consider. Since on-site clinics are typically small, you're often the only PT on duty. So you need to be comfortable working by yourself without any collegial interaction. Also, you likely won't have access to large or highly technical equipment at your clinic. When your treatment plan requires such equipment, you must refer the patient out.

Along those same lines, if a patient needs a treatment you aren't certified to provide—such as dry needling or manipulation—another team member won't be on hand to help. Again, you have to refer your patient. While PTs are used to referring out when needed, it does delay care. It also shines a light on gaps in your care abilities, and it never feels good to expose your shortcomings to the client.

If you have chosen to go into business for yourself (which you know I recommend), when you are sick or have a family emergency, you can't just call your supervisor. You are the supervisor. It's up to you to put in place a way to meet your contractual obligation to your client. This can mean finding and paying a qualified replacement to cover your shift or working out a plan with your client to work the weekend or different hours that week. I've found that if you have a good relationship with your client, covering rare emergencies is not a problem.

With on-site PT, often you are on your own. There is no executive entity to depend on or to pick up the slack when life happens to you. As a business owner and independent contractor, these everyday problems of running a business and caring for patients become yours to solve.

A BETTER WAY TO PRACTICE

It's rewarding to walk around the facility, production area, or warehouse where your clinic is located and see employees you've helped. It feels good when they stop you to ask questions about an ache or pain they've been having or some general medical issue that's been on their mind, or they show you a stressor they've identified in their work area and ask for your help in reporting it to the safety team. It feels extraordinarily useful to be a valued set of eyes and a different sort of lens for that corporate team.

The job of an on-site PT does come with more responsibility than being an employee at a brick-and-mortar clinic. But as you now know, it also involves more exciting work, more independence over how you practice, the ability to be proactive for your patients, and the opportunity to use your PT skills and your ingenuity in ways you didn't know were possible within the physical therapy profession.

What the job of on-site PT comes down to is making the world work better for people who work. And because of the way the on-site practice model works, we PTs benefit from this unique model of care as well.

....

EXERCISE
The Pros & Cons of On-Site PT for You

....

Questions

1. How does the on-site PT's mandate—prevention and wellness—change your thinking around your practice? For better or worse?

2. Do the expanded responsibilities and services of the on-site PT attract you? Repel you? Scare you? Excite you?

3. How do you feel about being able to see your patients regularly as they go about their day? How do you feel about getting to know them?

4. What part of the job of on-site PT do you think you'd enjoy the most and why?

5. What part of the job do you have the most doubts about, and why?

6. What part of your current job would you miss if you became an on-site PT?

7. How would your priorities be different as an on-site PT?

8. How do you see your life changing if you choose to become an on-site PT?

Activity

- Using the information above, write out your list of pros and cons about becoming an on-site PT.

3

―――

A DAY IN MY LIFE AS AN ON-SITE PT

The rhythm of your days is different in on-site practice as compared to a day at a brick-and-mortar clinic—as are your responsibilities. As a business owner and independent contractor, you must fit the varying demands of running a business along with the clinic work you've contracted for into each day. To give you an idea of what this might look like, here's an overview of a typical workday in my life as an on-site PT.

THE MORNING ROUTINE

Most days start in my home office. With a fresh cup of coffee in my hand and my dog snuggling beside me, I spend about thirty minutes working on my business before heading into the clinic.

Since I currently have contracts with three companies, and employ and place several on-site PTs (including myself) at their clinics, the first thing I do is check all my client email accounts. Since I can only physically be at one site each day, I use email to manage my employees, review their patient lists, and stay involved and informed in their activities. I may also need to answer emails about an employee's ability to return to work or RSVP to an online meeting with my client's operations or safety team to discuss injuries or a "near-miss" situation.

Weekly, I check my bank accounts to make sure invoices to my business have been paid. As a business owner who is responsible for my paycheck, as well as my employees' paychecks, making sure all invoices are paid on time is something I monitor closely.

Depending on what day of the week it is and which client site I've scheduled myself for, I either leave the house at 8:00 a.m. or 11:00 a.m. Occasionally, I work during a swing or overnight shift if requested by the client. This is infrequent, but I make it a standard offer in most contracts so my clients can be confident that all their employees are covered by my company's services, no matter what shift they work.

On days when I have a later start, I use the extra hours at home to get in a short workout, a longer dog walk, and a little more home-office time. I use that time to take care of things like payroll, personnel-required documentation, invoicing, and researching any new clinical practical guidelines or training required by my state or by my client.

Then I'm out the door to the clinic.

CLINIC TIME

The on-site PT clinic is a simple set up with a personalized, low-tech, movement-based approach to employee health. It is not expensive or labor intensive to set up an on-site PT clinic. I can work in just about any size space, as long as it has a treatment table. However, I do prefer that space is as close to the employee time clock or break room as possible. This facilitates regular contact with the employees. You want to see every employee every day when you are on the job.

Typically, the on-site clinic space varies based on what the client makes available. Right now, at one site, I have a 10 ft. x 10 ft. space with a treatment table. At another site, I have a 15 ft. x 30 ft. space, complete with a desk, stool, a treatment table, and some other basic clinic amenities like resistance bands, a few weights, heat packs, and ice packs. My third site is attached to a large gym—which gives me all kinds of room and equipment to work with.

Once I arrive on-site, I check with the safety department to see if there are any issues that need to be addressed immediately. If there are none, I walk the shop floor to check on employees and see if anyone who's not on that day's schedule needs to be.

My daily clinic volume typically ranges from four to ten patients. Even when it's ten, it's not as stressful as it was at the brick-and-mortar clinic because I know each patient and their issues well. I prioritize the appointment schedule for urgency and work-relatedness—always with the goal of minimizing the patient's time away from work.

A smooth clinic schedule rarely happens. The passage of time is not something employees hard at work on the floor focus on. Most of them work until they come to a good stopping point, and then they remember they had a PT appointment. When employees miss appointments or forget altogether—which is often—I go out on the floor, find them, and reschedule.

My patient sessions on-site look similar in some ways to a standard session at an outpatient clinic. If the person is at work and on the clock, my goal is to provide care with maximum impact in as little amount of time as possible, so they can return to work. Though if their issue calls for more time, I do not hesitate to take it. Typically, I do an evaluation, identify any red flags or contributory medical conditions, perform a relevant examination, perhaps apply manual and movement treatment. I use heat or ice if needed to reduce swelling or pain, general massage, and KT/athletic taping. I also discuss basic movement strategies. And before they leave my clinic, I schedule time to come to their station to watch them work, either that day or the next clinic day—to make sure their work movement is not creating or irritating their injury.

If someone is out of work or on light duty, I'll take a more comprehensive approach. If needed, we have a longer session—perhaps employing treatments such as full body strengthening, job simulation, conditioning, and an extensive home program.

When I have a break in my day, I use it to quickly check email, text, and phone messages from my staff. Though I'm at my client site, I'm still available to my staff should any issues arise, or they need me to problem-solve—though I am sensitive to only respond to them on my time.

PREVENTION

As you well know by now—and I'll continue to stress throughout this book—the job of the on-site PT is as much about prevention as it is about treatment. An important part of my workday is blocking time to be out of the clinic, observing employees at work, and looking for ways to prevent injuries. Sometimes I have no agenda. I simply observe. Sometimes I follow a current patient to learn what their job is or to watch their movement. Always, I use my floor time to remind employees about the on-site clinic and the services available to them.

I try to watch different employees do the same job and observe any differences in movement. I also ask about and document situations that can have an immediate impact on injury risk while working (such as slotting heavy items below shoulder height in a warehouse). I use various ergonomic screening tools to help find ergonomic risks and improve conditions.

When observing employees working, I make it a habit to remind myself that the employee is the expert at their job, not me. Before suggesting anything, it's extremely important to be educated by the person doing the job, to find out why they operate a certain way. Then, and only then, do I sparingly make suggestions based on ergonomic stressor findings. If I don't honor and appreciate the thousands of hours they've put into their job and just start shooting out ways for the employee to be better, I will not gain their trust and they will not respect my suggestions. Often, when I ask the right questions, employees can see the issue more fully than I can and find the best solution themselves intuitively.

TESTING

Not all clients have their on-site PTs perform post-offer, pre-employment testing (POET), although it is one of the most impactful services we can offer. I encourage my clients to take advantage of this service, because it can make a huge impact on hiring and safety costs right out of the gate.

I typically schedule around thirty to forty-five minutes for these tests, depending on the job the candidate has been offered. I do a quick musculoskeletal screen, then ask them to perform some of the tasks the position requires—such as lifting, bending, climbing stairs, carrying, or repetitive or dexterous hand work.

I also use this opportunity to instill the company's safety culture in these future employees. During the test, I focus on teaching good manual material handling methods. I also discuss job fitness and the overall wellness benefits of the company.

DAY'S END

As with all PT jobs, the day ends with documentation. I use a simple electronic medical records (EMR) system that allows me to document preventive care as well. There's no insurance billing to worry about with on-site care. (More on systems and equipment in Section III.)

I try to document during the day as I go, but I may need to spend thirty minutes once I'm back in my home office to finish notes, send a fax to a workers' compensation physician, or research a brace or a tool to help improve an employee's work comfort. I also make sure my clients are informed of the clinic schedule and any issues that arose that day. This generates trust and a willingness to be flexible on the rare occasion that an issue does arise. Again, I have figured this home-office time into my contracted fee, so it's compensated time.

The day goes fast. But I don't feel overwhelmed or overworked. After two decades as an on-site PT, I continue to find the work stimulating. Every day is an exercise in being well informed, operating from a position of excellence and honesty, and focusing on the employees and their wellness.

....

EXERCISE

Is On-Site PT the Way You Want to Spend Your Day?

....

Questions

1. What does the start of your day look like now? How do you see it changing if you become an on-site PT?

2. How do you feel about working part of your day from home—having duties outside your clinic time? Is it a pro or a con for you?

3. What did you find most appealing about my day? And why?

4. What did you find most concerning? And why?

5. Do you feel you have the patience to deal with patients forgetting their PT appointments? How would you handle this reality of on-site work?

6. Did anything in this chapter give you pause about becoming an on-site PT? Why? Is it a deal-breaker? Why or why not?

7. Are extra services—such as pre-employment testing—something you're interested in educating yourself about?

8. What is the end of your day like now? How does it compare to the end of my day?

9. As you learn more about on-site PT, is it becoming more or less attractive to you? Why or why not?

Activity

- Create a weekly schedule for what you think your on-site practice might look like based on the "typical" day described in this chapter. Compare it to your current weekly schedule. Note your thoughts.

Section Two

THE ON-SITE PT BUSINESS MODEL

If the job of the on-site PT has piqued your interest, your next step is understanding what exactly goes into a successful on-site practice and how to get those necessary elements into yours. Every successful business begins with a business model. Don't let that phrase—business model—throw you. It's simply a plan. It defines who your clients are, what services you offer, the type of business you're going to operate, and the steps you need to create the business.

Your business model for your on-site PT practice will be unique to you and the market you choose to serve. It will also grow and change to reflect your preferences as your business matures. This section provides you with the basics to consider as your business model takes shape.

4

THE ON-SITE CLIENT

The most important component in any business is the client. As a business owner, you must have in-depth knowledge of who your client is, your client's business goals, and the problems your client needs you to solve for them.

As we've discussed, as an on-site physical therapist, your client is most often the self-insured or self-funded company. Your patients are the employees of that company. But it's the self-insured company you contract with and the self-insured company that pays your invoices.

Therefore, it benefits you to understand how self-insurance works and why your clients choose it. It's also useful to appreciate the relationship between self-insurance and on-site care, and how you—the on-site PT—enhance the advantages of self-insuring for your clients. This deep understanding of your clients' motivations allows you to not only respond to your clients' needs with the necessary services but also to anticipate those needs and offer additional services.

HOW SELF-INSURANCE WORKS

With a traditional insurance policy (known in the industry as a "fully funded" plan), an employer buys a health care policy from an insurance company, and the insurance company assumes responsibility for paying all claims.

With a "self-funded" or "self-insured" plan, employers design their own health insurance policy (adhering to applicable government regulations), collect premiums themselves, and assume direct financial responsibility for paying their employees' medical claims. In most cases, self-insured employers hold all contributions and collected premiums in trust. When a claim needs to be paid, money is taken from that trust.

To be clear, these self-insured companies are not in the insurance business. Most manage the financial portion of health insurance themselves and utilize a third-party administrator (TPA) to manage the claims and administrate the services.

For the employees of self-insured companies, the user experience is much the same as with traditional insurance. The plan provides a list of available medical services and providers. There are co-pays, deductibles, maximum out-of-pocket values, and premiums that the employer and employee pay.

INSURING THE BOTTOM LINE

When I first accepted an on-site PT position, I didn't know it was possible for a company to self-insure and I didn't understand why a company would want to. I perceived self-insurance to be very expensive and difficult to administer. Why not just negotiate a good policy from a major insurance company and let them handle everything, including the risk?

A bit of research on insurance costs, premiums, and health care cost trends revealed the answer. Between 2000 and 2010, health care insurance premiums increased by an incredible 80 percent. In the last decade, they've increased another 55 percent. During those same years, company profits and employee salaries certainly did not increase at those same rates. Health insurance costs have created a heavy financial yoke for employees and employers alike. Today's employers are faced with the daunting task of providing health benefits to their employees without breaking the bank. You could argue that a primary fiscal liability—an actual risk for business—is the cost and volatility of health insurance premiums and the cost of health care itself. By self-insuring, employers rein in both those costs and their volatility.

According to the Self Insurance Education Foundation (SIEF), the overall financial benefit of self-funding insurance is decreased costs. The premium no longer must cover a traditional insurance company's overhead. It's no longer tied to a "per-claim" system in which the business can't predict how much health care their employees will need each year.

With self-insurance, the administration of the plan now comes under the employer's control, where all administration fees are set, stable, and smaller. The self-insured employer also saves on non-claim expenses, such as insurance commissions, risk charges, marketing, and state insurance premium taxes. All this not only saves money but also improves cash flow.

The major downsides of self-insuring are financial exposure and the considerable work involved in managing a plan. Fortunately, both have well-established solutions. Purchasing a stop-loss insurance policy reduces much of the financial exposure for the employer. These policies either limit the number of claims paid for each employee or limit the total amount paid for claims over the plan year. And as we've already discussed, hiring that TPA reduces the workload associated with implementing and managing self-insurance. These TPAs attend to some or all the details and day-to day-operations of the company's health-insurance plan.

So yes, the financial risk of self-insuring employee health care benefits is considerable. But, for companies with the necessary liquidity, the cost savings are well worth the risk. There are other benefits as well.

ENSURING FOCUSED HEALTH BENEFITS

In most cases, the self-insured company's health care policy meets the needs of the workforce better than a traditional policy—because the employer can design it to do so. As long as they keep to all applicable regulations, the self-insurer can pick and choose benefits and services—in an a-la-carte sort of way—to shape a health insurance package that fits their workforce. In contrast, when shopping for a fully funded plan, an employer can only choose from the packages the insurance provider offers. So companies often end up paying for benefits and services their employees don't need, sometimes to the exclusion of benefits they do.

Making their policies even stronger, the self-insured have access to all their claims data—information those with fully funded plans don't have access to. This claims information expands their ability to make effective health-plan modifications in a time-sensitive, fiscally responsible manner. By mining claims data, self-insurers can identify patterns and trends in employee health and benefit usage, and then can adjust their health plan accordingly.

The self-insurer also gets a break when it comes to regulation. Traditional insurers must follow both federal and state regulations when setting up and administering employer-sponsored health insurance plans. While federal laws are uniform throughout the country, state laws, of course, are unique to each state. Thus, a national business with a traditionally funded plan ends up with different coverage from state to state—making the plan more cumbersome to implement. Self-insured companies are exempt from state laws thanks to the Employment Retirement Income Security Act of 1974 (ERISA). This allows them to provide consistent health care benefits nationwide to all their employees, regardless of where they are located.

SELF-INSURING PAVES THE WAY FOR ON-SITE CARE

Because they foot the bill for their employees' health care costs, self-insured companies are incentivized to keep their workforce healthy. They stay on top of their employees' health status and needs. They also put a big focus on early treatment and prevention—making on-site care especially attractive to these companies. These employers regard on-site care as an investment toward fewer claims and lower insurance expenses overall—and as with any investment, they expect a return.

The on-site clinic—where you work—exists to deliver that return by preventing injury; eliminating wait times for care when an injury does occur; and avoiding excessive claims costs related to provider referrals, repeat visits, and insurance processes that are not a value add to the patient's health. No longer hindered by insurance company algorithms and approval procedures, your clients expect their on-site practices to be efficient—to evaluate patients immediately, treat them on-site when possible, or get them to the off-site care they need in an expedited manner.

In a traditionally insured company with no on-site PT clinic, for instance, a worker who arrives for his shift with a painful shoulder would be sent to see his family doctor to get a work release. The physician might provide medication and then recommend the employee attend PT (most insurance requires conservative care before imaging can be done.) It will take at least a couple of days to get a PT appointment. Not to mention, there may be a delay for the insurance authorization. Then, after four to six therapy sessions, this employee will go back to the doctor for evaluation. If their condition hasn't improved, an MRI authorization may be requested, which usually takes another week. Once the MRI is completed, the employee—and the employer—must wait on another appointment with the physician to interpret it.

This employee might be unable to work this whole time. If they do report to work with a painful shoulder with limited mobility, a physician or PT can't monitor them because the PT is off-site. The employee's work output may suffer, and they could further injure themself. Neither of these scenarios will turn out well for the employee or the company.

When that same employee works at a company with an on-site clinic, if they report to work with pain, they're sent to the clinic immediately. The PT screens them for any serious shoulder injury. If the findings are benign, the PT provides preventative care: basic movement suggestions, self-care education, ice, taping, and general massage, if appropriate. If the PT determines that specific treatment is warranted, they provide it immediately right there (subject to the direct-access laws of the state). The expense and time lost to the employee and the company are minimal. If the PT suspects serious injury, they send the employee to a physician with a detailed note, which expedites the process of getting the care or imaging needed. (In some cases, the PT can order imaging—again, subject to state regulation.)

The on-site PT, safety representative, and the employee then discuss if the employee can return to work immediately or should take a day or two off to rest the shoulder. Whenever the employee does return to work, the on-site PT ensures they receive daily preventive care and any treatment needed to help them continue to heal. Further, the PT observes the employee's working habits to ensure safe practices to prevent further aggravation of the injury.

No matter the severity or type of injury, the on-site option produces better outcomes for the employer, the employee, and the treatment provider.

Historically, self-insurance has made the most financial sense for larger companies with reliable revenue sources and a good-size workforce (two hundred or more). Self-insurance—and on-site clinics that come with it—are especially attractive to enterprises where on-the-job injuries are more likely to occur, such as companies that deal in transportation and material handling, health care, maintenance, production, distribution, construction, and extraction industries. Think about who those companies might be in your own community. Some well-known leaders in on-site employee wellness and injury prevention programs include Tesla, Amazon, Toyota, and Chevron.

THE SELF-INSURED COMPANY—OUR CLIENT—IS HERE TO STAY

As health insurance premiums continue to climb, self-insuring is making more sense for more companies. It's a trend on the rise—meaning your client pool is on the rise too. According to the Kaiser Family Foundation's 2020 Employee Benefits Survey, 67 percent of covered workers overall and 84 percent of covered workers in bigger organizations are enrolled in self-insured plans. A percentage that's increased since 2019 and translates into approximately one hundred and fifty million workers currently being covered this way.

Most important for physical therapists and the growth of on-site practices, self-insured companies realize and appreciate the value of wellness. They know that by maximizing the benefits of self-insurance and on-site care, they reap a return that goes well beyond an insurance policy.

EXERCISE:
Fully Understanding Your Role in Self-Insurance

Questions

1. How do you feel in general about self-insurance? Is it something you are familiar with?
2. Can you explain to yourself why self-insurance is a sound insurance instrument for larger companies?
3. What surprises you, if anything, about the number and type of companies that self-insure?
4. What attracts you most about working for a self-insured company?
5. What concerns you most about working for a self-insured company?
6. How do you see self-insurance as affecting your work as an on-site PT? What do you need to be prepared to do that you don't do in your current position?
7. What responsibilities does self-insurance allow you to let go of as a PT?
8. How do you feel about being relied on as an expert and a problem-solver in the areas of wellness and prevention?

Activity

- Go to the Self Insurance Education Foundation (SIEF) (http:// www.siefonline.org) to learn more about self-funded insurance and get ideas for how on-site PT can add value to your clients' operations.

5

OSHA, WORKERS' COMP, AND ON-SITE PT SERVICES

Our clients themselves are not versed in the intricacies of effective health care application. They contract with us—an outside licensed professional service—for that expertise. They look to us as PTs to translate their health, wellness, and safety goals into measurable gains via the on-site clinic. They rely on us to educate them as to the best way to keep their employees healthy. We advise them on which measures will best promote safety and continually improve their on-site health services. We keep their costs in check through prevention. When we need to treat their employees, we do so efficiently and get them back to work. We are an important part of the wellness and safety culture for their workforce. Our proactive approach makes us instrumental to their company's mission.

All this places a significant burden of responsibility on on-site PTs, which we need to be more than capable of handling. A common sentiment of on-site care is that it positively affects employees from the hiring date to retiring date. Every day on the job can and does bring a new challenge and a new opportunity for us to show our expertise to our clients and our patients through the services we offer.

BUILDING ON YOUR PT EXPERTISE

One afternoon while on-site, I was called to attend a safety team meeting. We had a problem—a recent increase in lower-back strains in the plant's production areas. The incidents were significant enough that they were considered a recordable injury by the Occupational Safety and Health Administration (OSHA). They would also lead to an increase in workers' compensation claims. Our team was tasked with finding the root cause(s) of these injuries and minimizing the risk before workers' compensation claims climbed and OSHA flagged the plant for a safety audit.

During our investigation, the employees reported more difficulty and stress than before when lifting boxes onto the packaging machine. As it turns out, the supplier that provided these packaging materials had increased the box size and weight to save money on transportation costs. From the supplier's perspective, this change made great sense. Being able to fit a few more boxes on a pallet can save a company millions of dollars annually. But on the receiving end (our end), their small changes were creating more physical stress on our workers—and so adding to our costs.

These boxes, which our employees had to lift from a pallet to a conveyor, had increased from thirty-five pounds to forty-two pounds. If an employee was lifting approximately two boxes per minute over an average shift, this meant they were lifting more than a thousand "extra" pounds per shift. This change in weight was creating more physical stress on our employees, leading to reports of low-back injury, more lost time from work, more OSHA-recordable cases, and more workers' compensation claims.

We could not change the weight of the boxes provided by our supplier. But we could change how our employees moved and the time they spent performing that task. Therefore, our challenge became what movement and time span exactly would eliminate injury while assuring the necessary productivity?

There were multiple suggestions from the assembled safety team. From my own ergonomic toolbox, I recommended we use the National Institute for Occupational Safety and Health (NIOSH) lifting equation to ensure whatever plan we came up with would work. After experimenting with various combinations of box-lift heights, distances the boxes would be carried, number of people at the station, and time spent performing that job task, we were able to determine the right arrangement to reduce the stressors on our workers and prevent injury. Once we put these modifications in place, we got the results we'd calculated for. OSHA-recordable injuries and workers' compensation claims due to low-back injuries vanished in this work area.

In your transition to on-site care, treating individual patients may remain the central hub of the services you provide. But it will be your ability to intervene to prevent injury across the facility and reduce the consequences (physical and financial) of injuries that will be seen as the most valuable services you provide by your patients and clients alike. Patients will look to you to keep them working. Clients will look to you to help them improve safety on the job and maintain compliance.

As a practicing PT, you already have the skills to figure out root causes of injury and determine solutions for prevention. From the time you entered PT school, you were trained to watch a person move, identify stressed areas on the body, and teach improvements. These things likely come naturally to you now. Your knowledge of ergonomic tools—like the NIOSH lifting equation—further allows you to quantify the risks and devise solutions.

To expand your services in this area and become indispensable to clients, you also need to maintain an up-to-date understanding of safety culture and safety regulations, such as OSHA and workers' comp. You must know what they are, how they work, and how you can use them to their best advantage for your patients and clients. Such services are key to your on-site success.

THE RULES & REGS THAT GOVERN YOUR SERVICES

Wisely, most companies have strong policies and procedures related to safety. They have safety teams and a safety representative to both generate and enforce those policies and procedures. They invest in safety training for employees. They maintain processes to consistently review and update their efforts. Some even make "safety" a company value and put their commitment to it in their mission statement. They want to make sure that everyone, from new hires to the CEO, understands that safety holds a top spot on the company's hierarchy of performance measures. Taken together, all these actions add up to their "safety culture."

Hiring you, an on-site PT, is another demonstration of their commitment. While the values, protocols, and procedures help define the safety culture, it's your boots on the ground (your work one-on-one with employees) that help employees understand and commit to safety on an individual, personal level.

Government regulations and requirements—mainly administered by OSHA and workers' compensation—drive every US company's safety culture. Therefore, these entities direct the services you offer and the way you work, as well.

OSHA, a federal agency under the Department of Labor, mandates a variety of industry safety standards to protect employees. It also requires documentation from the company of any workplace safety accidents or injuries that necessitate medical care. The incidents are recorded in the

OSHA 300 log. Workers' compensation is an insurance system governed by each state. It provides compensation to employees who lose wages or have medical expenses due to a work-related injury or illness. All states require businesses to have workers' compensation insurance in some form and require filing a claim for medical costs and/or time lost due to work-related injuries.

The company-sponsored health insurance and the workers' compensation insurance are two different policies and are mutually exclusive of each other. However, companies who self-insure for health care may (and often do) also choose to go the self-funded route with their workers' compensation policy—meaning they take on financial liability for their workers' comp claims. Most states require that the workers' compensation policy be administered by a qualified carrier. Self-insured companies can meet this requirement by contracting with a TPA that is also a qualified workers' comp carrier.

Penalties for noncompliance with either OSHA or workers' compensation are substantial—and to be avoided. A high number of workers' compensation claims can trigger higher premiums, lower worker morale, and translate into a poor insurability rating for the employer. Companies with a large number of OSHA-recordable incidents, violations of OSHA standards, or failures to comply (monitored by OSHA) can find themselves with increased OSHA oversight, audits, and fines. They can also experience an onslaught of unfavorable news stories, which lead to bad public and investor relations. You might remember a meatpacking plant being shut down for ten days in 2020 due to OSHA violations. The violations cost the company millions of dollars in fines and lost revenue. They also made headlines across the country. But the real bottom line for any company here is that standards are put in place to avoid serious workplace injury and/or illnesses. Failure to comply can and often does lead to serious injury to workers.

A well-informed on-site PT can help protect their clients from unnecessary reporting, excessive claims, needless penalties, and harm to their workers. These are all areas that your on-site services can make a real difference for your clients and make you invaluable.

THE PT AS GATEKEEPER

When we worked in a brick-and-mortar clinic, we witnessed the results of on-the-job injuries and safety problems. As on-site PTs, we become safety gatekeepers, working to prevent harm and minimize any injury's effects for our patients and clients.

Typically, the on-site PT is first on the scene when an employee reports an injury or illness. We are first to hear the employee's version of events. We are first to evaluate the issue. And we propose the course of treatments. While we don't ultimately make the call when it comes to regulation compliance, reporting, or claims—the company's safety representative does that—how we document the incident, identify the problem, and choose the care provided greatly informs that decision.

To serve the situation honestly and appropriately for our patients and client, we must understand how our words and actions are interpreted through the lens of safety culture and the regulatory agencies involved. For instance, you must know that having pain or discomfort at work and having an injury that is "work-related" are two different things. And you must know how to describe both correctly in your documentation.

Fortunately, much of what the on-site PT needs to know to skillfully navigate the regulatory world can be found through understanding seven terms—OSHA- Recordable, First Aid, Report Only, Treatment-Medical Care, Medical Only Claim, Indemnity Claim, and Lost Time (as defined by either OSHA or workers' compensation):

OSHA-Recordable

On its website (osha.gov/recordkeeping), OSHA defines a recordable injury or illness as:

- Any work-related fatality.
- Any work-related injury or illness that results in loss of consciousness, days away from work, restricted work, or transfer to another job.
- Any work-related injury or illness requiring medical treatment beyond first aid.
- Any work-related diagnosed case of cancer, chronic irreversible diseases, fractured or cracked bones or teeth, and punctured eardrums.
- There are also special recording criteria for work-related cases involving: needlesticks and sharps injuries; medical removal; hearing loss; and tuberculosis.

First Aid (OSHA)

Again, on its website (www.osha.gov/medical-first-aid/recognition), OSHA defines first aid as quick, immediate medical attention delivered on the spot and not requiring specific medical skills. The OSHA website gives examples of first aid as ". . . cleaning minor cuts, scrapes, or scratches; treating a minor burn; applying bandages and dressings; the use of nonprescription medicine; draining blisters; removing debris from the eyes; massage; and drinking fluids to relieve heat stress."

Knowing what OSHA considers first aid allows you to provide more precise and useful documentation to the company's safety representative. As long as the employee can perform 100 percent of their job duties with no physician-ordered restrictions after receiving first aid, the incident is not considered a recordable injury under OSHA.

Report Only (OSHA)

When an incident does not meet the requirements to trigger an OSHA recordable (i.e., you find no need for formal medical care and no lost time from work/restricted duty), it is deemed "report only." This means the incident is reported only to the safety team. The takeaway here for you is that when a formal report to OSHA or the workers' compensation insurance carrier is not required, you (the on-site PT) must still "report" the injury to the company's safety team and document the care you provided through your clinic records.

Treatment-Medical Care (OSHA)

Again, in OSHA-speak, this phrase refers to treatment that is specific to a diagnosis, is ongoing, and requires professional training to apply—such as rigid splinting, location-specific massage, or skilled physical therapy interventions. Such treatment would need to be reported to the safety department for the purpose of OSHA reporting.

Medical Only Claim (Workers' Comp)

This phrase refers specifically to a claim submitted to workers' compensation. If it's determined by the safety representative that an employee has had an on-the-job injury and the employee receives medical treatment that involves a cost, a First Report of Injury (FROI) must be submitted to the workers' comp insurance carrier to initiate a claim.

Just a note here regarding workers' compensation claims: Always keep in mind when seeing an injured employee that first aid measures (as defined by OSHA) are not recordable or considered treatment, so no workers' compensation claim is submitted. If you provide diagnosis-specific care or care that requires a skilled provider, then you have initiated treatment, and the case becomes a workers' compensation claim. If the patient's situation falls somewhere between calling for first aid and initiating treatment, you can provide the first aid care and then refer the patient to the client's workers' compensation provider to determine if further treatment is required. That way the employee gets some first aid care and education on their condition before seeing the physician.

Indemnity Claim (Workers' Comp)

Another aspect of workers' comp, an indemnity claim reimburses the injured employee for lost wages. A workers' compensation claim becomes an "indemnity claim" when an employee loses a specified amount of time at work due to a work-related "medical claim." However, each state determines how much time must be lost before a claim is considered a lost time claim. In Colorado, for example, the employee must miss three regular shifts before the claim becomes an indemnity claim.

Lost Time (OSHA)

With OSHA, "lost time" refers to any and all time an employee cannot perform their normal job duties because of a work-related injury. This term is different from the workers' compensation indemnity claim's "lost time." For example, in Colorado, while missing two shifts won't qualify as an indemnity claim, it will be considered "lost time" for OSHA and needs to be reported as such.

These two definitions of "lost time" provide you with a frame of what each agency is looking for and counting. Where workers' compensation is looking to make the worker whole again financially, OSHA is keeping data on actual workplace injuries and their consequences. Both agencies use such data to improve workplace safety for everyone.

Two other terms you might run into when reviewing a company's entire safety record are DART (days away, restricted, or transferred) levels and TRIR (total recordable incident rates). Calculating these is beyond your responsibility as an on-site PT, but it's good to know what they mean.

The chart below shows how a wrist sprain would be categorized, using the terms above, based upon the type of intervention applied:

Event: Wrist Sprain On-the-Job Injury	Safety Team Helps Employee	Sent to offsite Physician For Exam, Deemed First Aid Only	Sent to Offsite Physician for Exam	Sent to On-Site PT for Exam	Sent to On-Site PT for Exam	Sent to On-Site PT for Exam
	Elastic Wrap Applied	Soft Brace Applied	Rigid Brace Applied	Soft Brace Applied	Rigid Brace Applied	Rigid Brace Applied
	Returned to Work	Returned to Work	Returned to Work	Returned to Work	Returned to Work	Returned to Work Day 2
Internal Report Only	✓			✓		
OSHA-Recordable			✓		✓	✓
OSHA Lost time						✓
First Aid Case	✓	✓		✓		
Workers Comp Medical Claim		✓	✓			
Workers Comp Indemnity Claim						

For instance, say an employee slips on the job. As the on-site PT, you determine immediately that they've broken their arm and refer them for off-site care. They initially miss a week of work. Then they return to lighter duty until their arm is healed and the cast can be removed.

Every detail of this incident goes in your clinic report. Taking into account the medical care provided and the financial expenditure for that care, this would be a recordable and lost-time injury. It would need to be reported to OSHA. In most states, it would also qualify to be filed with the company's workers' compensation carrier since there was medical cost associated with the care provided and the employee missed multiple shifts at work.

Say a different employee slips at work. This time, the result is a sprained wrist. You, as the on-site PT, determine that first aid care (as defined by OSHA) is all that's needed in this instance. You treat the employee with ice, athletic taping, general movement for the upper extremity, and give them instructions on how to care for their sprain. The employee returns to work immediately. When you check on them later, you assess their work ability, look for any ergonomic or safety issues, and offer solutions to some minor issues you see that can be easily corrected with administrative or behavior controls.

In this second scenario, there were no formal medical interventions or costs, no treatment outside of first aid, no lost time as defined by either OSHA or workers' comp. You keep a detailed report of this for the PT clinic. Based on that report, chances are that the safety administrator will find no need to report to either OSHA or workers' comp on this employee incident.

In both these scenarios not only did you provide accurate documentation of these workplace incidents, but in the second scenario you limited external costs for your clients. If the employee in that scenario had been sent off-site to be seen by a doctor (i.e., have medical care with a fee attached), the company would have had no choice but to file a report with

OSHA and submit a workers' compensation claim. Additionally, it is unlikely the employee would have returned to his regular job that same day, which triggers a lost-time recordable and adds indemnity to the claim.

If the treatment the worker received from the off-site provider falls within the "first aid" definition, it does not have to be reported to OSHA. It will, however, still generate a workers' compensation claim. If the employee returns for their next shift with no restrictions, there is no lost time. Our on-site services get the patient to the right place for care sooner than would happen using a nurse call line or off-site practitioner. We streamline the entire incident for both our patients and clients—so as not to waste anyone's time or money. We cut the red tape. We avoid outside intervention when possible. And when not possible, we send the client to the appropriate medical provider with notes, so they can receive care as quickly and effectively as possible. Even if an incident triggers an OSHA recordable, our on-site efforts still lower the cost of workers' compensation claims.

Of course, all injuries must go through proper reporting and an investigation process before being deemed "work related" or "OSHA reportable." But you can see how the on-site PT's immediate actions, accurate documentation, and professional opinions guide the investigation and influence that final decision.

KNOW THE LAWS—ALL OF THEM

OSHA and workers' comp rules and regulations aren't static. Neither are the laws that govern our PT practice. Therefore, it's a professional priority of the on-site PT to keep current with state and federal agencies that impact how we work, the services we can offer, as well as our client's compliance. This isn't as hard as it used to be. Much of what we need to know can be found and monitored online.

The place to start is the American Physical Therapy Association's website (www.apta.org). There you'll find resources for learning about licensure and compliance, including links for national programs such as the Health Insurance Portability and Accountability Act (HIPAA), workers' compensation information by states, and individual state regulatory boards. To learn more about OSHA and increase your knowledge of workplace injury and reporting skills, check out the educational trainings at https://www.osha.gov.

As you do the research into state laws affecting your practice, be sure to look into direct-access laws. As we talked about in Chapter 1, direct access means a patient can receive physical therapy treatments without first securing a physician's referral. All fifty states have some form of direct access for physical therapy, but some states have limitations and provisions on that access. Even in states that have full direct access, occasionally an insurance plan will require a physician's referral for services—though with self-insured plans this is not much of a concern.

What can be your concern, however, is in some states, workers' compensation requires a referral, even if the company is self-insured. You can see what the details of direct-access laws are in your state at https://www.apta.org/advocacy/issues/direct-access-advocacy/direct-access-by-state.

In those states with unrestricted direct access, not needing a physician referral has been a game changer for the on-site PT. Employees can come to you without any gatekeeper, time away from work, or expense. Not to mention that many studies over the years (and common sense) have concluded that early detection and intervention are advantageous to faster and fuller recoveries from injury.

For those states with provisional direct access, the on-site model still works well. The on-site PT can continue to be the first care provider, identify the patient's clinical diagnosis, and begin delivering care. You may need to get a physician referral after a certain number of visits or for a specific treatment (i.e., dry needling), but you can find ways to limit the barriers in between the employee and receiving care.

Regardless of the direct-access status, being on-site provides a great solution for patient noncompliance. When a patient doesn't follow up as ordered, you can go find them in the work area. Seeking that employee out sends a strong message that you care about them—which can encourage both compliance for that employee as well as increased on-site clinic utilization for that employee and their coworkers.

Imaging is another treatment area that's state regulated. Though being able to authorize imaging is relatively new for PTs, studies already show that we order it more sparingly and more appropriately than general practitioners for musculoskeletal conditions. As of this writing, there are only three states that allow PTs to order imaging—Colorado, Wisconsin, and Utah. Like with direct-access laws, more states are likely to come on board soon. You can keep up with all changes and advances to imaging laws at www.apta.org/patient-care/interventions/imaging.

SAFETY IS ITS OWN REWARD

Of all the PT skills I have, the services I provide in support of my client's safety culture are some of the most professionally and personally rewarding. They open all sorts of opportunities to be proactive for our patients, as you can see from this list of the most common safety-support services we provide:

- Educating employees as to how to move more safely and comfortably.
- Calling attention to hazards.

- Discussing general health issues and empowering employees.
- Letting management know what's helpful for their workers, what may be harming them, and what the company can change for the better.

By our very presence on-site, we help to build labor relations by being proof to workers that management cares about their well-being. While the services we offer our clients do save them money, make their workforce more productive, and keep the company in compliance with regulatory agencies, they also improve the health of the employees—our patients—every day, on the job and off.

After you've been on-site for a while, doing what you do best, you'll likely notice a kind of organic drive among employees—when the "safety magic" takes hold. The employees you've educated begin to spot movement problems for themselves and correct them before injuries happen. When they can't figure out what to do, they don't hesitate to call you to their worksite to analyze their movement. They freely ask questions of you and seek treatment for a "discomfort." They now understand it makes sense to see smaller pains as warning signs and not ignore them. When this "magic" starts, morale lifts, and safety naturally becomes even more embedded in how things are done in the company's culture. I've seen it happen many times—and you will too.

EXERCISE:
On-Site Services and Safety Protocols

Questions

1. How do safety culture and safety regulations figure into your current job?
2. What have you learned about on-the-job injury in your current PT practice that can inform your on-site practice?
3. How do you feel about participating in your clients' safety culture and compliance with safety regulations? Does the increased responsibility excite you or scare you or both? Why?
4. What current knowledge and skills can you add to a safety team? List them.

Activities

- Make flashcards of the OSHA and workers' comp terms in this chapter. Learn them inside and out, backward, and forward.
- Once you learn the terms, challenge yourself to use them in different patient scenarios you encounter in your current position. If you were an on-site PT, how would you report your patient's injury and why? How does your way of treating and reporting benefit your client?

Learn more about the laws that govern your on-site practice. Go to:

- American Physical Therapy Association's website (www.apta.org) for general information on licensure, compliance, and direct-access laws, as well as links to various regulatory boards and national programs.

- OSHA website (www.osha.gov) for trainings on workplace injury and reporting skills.
- Make a plan for staying current with OSHA and workers' comp regulations, as well as your clients' safety culture.

6

———

UNDERSTAND YOUR WORTH

Foundational to your business plan—underlying both your client's decision to invest in you and your decision on what services to offer—is value. We've discussed value—knowing intuitively that we make a real difference in the workplace. However, for value to be tangible and useful to a business, it must be measurable. Potential clients and current clients will have difficulty recognizing the cost savings that you—their on-site PT—deliver. Therefore, it's your job to provide any current or potential clients with the clinical, safety, and financial data to see your services as invaluable to their operation. Providing that evidence in dollars and cents will make current and potential clients sit up and pay attention to you every time.

Translating the services you offer into cost savings for the balance sheet allows all interested parties to better understand your contribution as an on-site PT. The data you provide informs your shared vision for the on-site clinic services, clarifies expectations, and keeps everyone on track as the clinic and your business evolve. In addition, these calculations are always welcomed by the person who must approve a budget and financial plan for the on-site PT services. Having real-time monitoring and cost-saving calculations makes their job easier. Not to mention, this data can be used for monthly key performance indicators (KPI) reporting and is instrumental in renegotiating your contract.

THE SUM OF YOUR WORTH

The cost of on-the-job injury can be broken down into two areas: clinical and safety. You can use those same two areas to calculate the dollar value of your on-site PT services. For your purposes, "clinical" emphasizes the value added by keeping care on-site by triaging possible injuries and providing OSHA-defined first aid. "Safety" emphasizes the cost savings related to injury prevention, employee hiring and retention, and ongoing condition management for employees in the work areas.

Within these two areas, you can leverage direct and indirect costs to get the best estimate on the cost savings you deliver. The Coordinating Committee for Automotive Repair (CCAR) is an organization that offers safety and environmental best-practices training (among other things) for the automotive industry worldwide. CCAR has a great blog describing what direct and indirect costs should be considered when calculating the costs of an on-the-job injury (https://ccar-greenlink.org/so-what-does-it-cost-a-company-when-someone-gets-hurt-on-the-job/). According to the blog, direct costs are things that may seem obvious with a lost-time injury and include:

- Medical costs
- Disability or indemnity payments
- Any program costs, such as claims management.

Indirect costs are not so apparent but are very real for the employer. They include:

- Wages paid to absent workers
- Wage costs related to time lost through work stoppage associated with the worker injury
- Overtime costs necessitated by an injury
- Administrative time spent by supervisors, safety personnel, and clerical workers after an injury
- Training costs for a replacement worker
- Cost of an insurance premium increase
- Lost productivity
- Clean-up, repair, and replacement costs from damaged material, machinery, property, and production errors.

According to the CCAR blog post, as a general guide, indirect costs surprisingly end up being equal to the direct costs for cases of more than $10,000 (which many cases are), so a 1:1 ratio. In other words, if someone requires $30,000 of care, then the total costs (direct + indirect) to the company would be approximately $60,000.

That might sound high, but when someone must seek medical care due to a work injury, costs add up quickly. Not only does outside care involve a lot of people, but the costs to cover the employee's work are also significant. Because these indirect costs are not usually covered by insurance, they have a direct impact on the company and its bottom line.

Tracking the injury data and cases of injury avoidance allows your clients to see exactly where you, the on-site PT, add value through cost savings—and where not having your services is going to cost them. It can also reveal areas that might need more attention, areas for which you can justify and propose additional services.

MAKING YOUR CLINICAL CASE

Study after study supports physical therapy as the preferred first line of treatment for musculoskeletal injury—the most common type of on-the-job injury. Seeing a physical therapist first produces better outcomes and fewer costs up front, as well as in the long run.

As an example, lower-back pain (LBP) is the number one musculoskeletal reason people visit their physician. Medicine spends more than $100 billion a year trying to alleviate this common and elusive pain. Medical treatment protocols routinely use imaging early in the course of care with the treating physician.

However, a 2015 study found that when the MRI is the first step in treating LBP, the overall cost of treatment increased more than 70 percent as compared to when physical therapy is the first intervention provided. (Fritz JM, Brennan GP, Hunter SJ. *Physical Therapy or Advanced Imaging as First Management Strategy Following a New Consultation for Low Back Pain in Primary Care: Associations with Future Health Care Utilization and Charges.* Health Serv Res. 2015 Dec; 50(6):1927-40.)

Bolstering those findings, a 2020 report from the Workers' Compensation Research Institute found that patients who received PT more than thirty days after reporting LBP had treatment costs that were 25 percent higher than patients receiving PT within thirty days. The same study found that those who had delayed entrance to PT had 58 to 69 percent more time in disability than those who received physical therapy earlier. (Wang D, Mueller K, and Lea R, *The Timing of Physical Therapy for Low Back Pain: Does It Matter in Workers' Compensation?* September 2020. WC-20-25.)

Still a third study from a military health system found that if a patient received PT within fourteen days of reporting LBP to a physician, that patient's treatment costs were lowered by 60 percent over a two-year follow-up period. These same patients' medical costs were lower overall, suggesting the benefits of physical therapy extended beyond their primary reason for seeking treatment and benefited their general health. (Childs JD, Fritz JM, Wu SS, Flynn TW, Wainner RS, Robertson EK, Kim FS, George SZ. Erratum to: *Implications of Early and Guideline Adherent Physical Therapy for Low Back Pain on Utilization and Costs.* BMC Health Serv Res. 2016 Aug 26; 16(1):444.)

Such studies helped me see where to look within my own clinic and services for procedures that would easily allow me to quantify my value. We want our clients to see in real-money terms what their costs might have been had they not had an on-site PT available.

MAKING YOUR SAFETY CASE

When it comes to the safety areas of our practice (prevention, monitoring, consulting), our value is best quantified by looking through two lenses: 1) The cost savings related to preventing an injury altogether. 2) The cost of disease and injury management as seen in patterns of absenteeism and presenteeism.

Absenteeism is defined as employees missing work beyond what's typical (occasional illness) and scheduled (paid time off). In general, chronic absenteeism adds stress to the workforce. It creates extra problems for those who are present, lowers morale, and increases fatigue. All that adds up to lower productivity, disruption of distribution schedules, and increased safety issues—costing the company money. Not to mention, the company may still have to pay an employee who is not there and not working, depending on the issue.

Presenteeism occurs when an employee is at work but not fully functional because of illness, injury, or psychological stressors. As with absenteeism, presenteeism results in lower productivity but with even more likelihood of increased accidents. When someone isn't operating at full capacity, they're more likely to make mistakes. Mistakes result in a higher probability of workplace accidents, putting everyone's safety at risk. Also a consideration, having an employee work through a chronic medical condition or injury can result in further aggravating the issue, causing higher medical bills or disability over time. In terms of illness, the employee may spread it to others and cause increased absenteeism or presenteeism.

According to the Community Wellbeing Index, presenteeism is estimated to cost United States employers $226 billion annually in lost productive time. Absenteeism is estimated to cost $84 billion annually. Absenteeism and presenteeism directly impact safety in the workplace and the company's bottom line. Companies are well aware of how much these conditions cost them.

CALCULATING THE COST OF AN INJURY

Now you know which factors to consider when making your financial case and the costs those factors typically place on a business. Next, you need to put a client's particular safety issue into dollars and cents. Luckily, OSHA's website has a calculator that makes it easy to figure out the financial ramifications of any injury.

The OSHA Safety-Pays Estimator (https://www.osha.gov/safetypays/estimator) assesses the whole cost—both direct and indirect—of on-the-job injuries. You can use it to show the cost saving (thus the value) of your on-site clinic treatments and your safety services (consulting, prevention, and monitoring) over a month, a quarter, a year, or whatever period of time you choose.

To show you how, let's look at the employee from the last chapter with the sprained wrist. To calculate my value to the company in caring for that injury, I would find my notes and plug the information into the OSHA Safety-Pays Estimator. Then I'd let the calculator determine the estimated costs of the injury had that employee been treated off-site by a physician.

Here's what that looks like:

Injury Type	Sprain
or	**OR**
Workers' Compensation Costs *(annual sum of costs)*	
Enter Profit Margin (%) *(leave blank to use default of 3%)*	3%
Enter Number of Injuries *(leave blank to use default of one)*	

Using default 3% Profit Margin

Estimated Total Cost

The extent to which the employer pays the direct costs depends on the nature of the employer's workers' compensation insurance policy. The employer always pays the indirect costs.

Injury Type	Instances	Direct Cost	Indirect Cost	Total Cost	Additional Sale (Indirect)	Additional Sale (Total)
Sprain	1	$30,487	$33,535	$64,022	$1,117,856	$2,134,066

Totals

Estimated Direct Costs:	$30,487
Estimated Indirect Costs:	$33,535
Combined Total (Direct and Indirect Costs):	$64,022
Sales to Cover Indirect Costs:	$1,1117,856
Sales to Cover Total Costs:	$2,134,066

Used with permission from OSHA and the National Council on Compensation Insurance, Inc. All rights reserved.

In this case, preventing one acute or repetitive strain injury from needing outside care saves the company $30,000 to $60,000. Now, multiply that by the number of sprains you treat on-site each year, as well as those you prevent altogether through your monitoring of employees' movements, and you have some powerful evidence of the value your on-site care services provide to the company.

Another point of value is the savings resulting from PT treatments provided on-site. Remember, if an employee had to go to an insurance-approved clinic, your client would be responsible for the cost of the medical claim. Let's say the average insurance reimbursement for a PT session is $140, and your contracted rate is $60 an hour as an on-site PT. For every treatment you provide, you save the company $80. You can gather information about allowable dollar amounts for each CPT code that you regularly utilize. (Research your state's workers' compensation medical fee schedule to determine allowable amounts for CPT codes.) Then you will have actual dollar values from which you can calculate unrealized costs (or cost savings). Equally valuable is the high-quality, one-on-one care and the positive employee experience it fosters.

SHOWING YOUR WORK AND YOUR VALUE

As you grow your on-site practice, the records you keep are paramount to boosting your business and showcasing this foundational element of your business. Use that information to calculate the cost of all the injuries and illnesses you treat and prevent. Then provide your clients with this objective data.

Do this on a regular basis—I recommend monthly—and you give them all the evidence they need to justify their investment in your on-site services. As a bonus, this information will be at your fingertips when it comes time to renegotiate your contract.

At the end of every pitch and negotiation, I remind my clients of a profound fact: *When you do not have on-site care of any kind, all the money you spend for medical and workers' compensation claims related to MSK injuries is spent outside the company, after the injury occurs. It makes sense to bring some of that care upstream, where the cost is less and you have the opportunity to prevent injuries in the first place.*

This is a true and powerful statement, and one you should be sure all your potential clients understand.

EXERCISE:
Show Your Value

Questions

1. How do you feel about breaking down your work into dollars and cents? Does it feel like it lessens what you do? Does it feel empowering?

2. Can you understand how this information helps clients to see how important your on-site care is to their operation?

3. Can you see how knowing your value in dollars and cents can support your negotiations for upgrading your services and equipment and increasing your own salary when the time comes?

Activities

- Learn more about the various factors that can go into calculating the cost of injury to businesses at the CCAR (https://ccar-green-link.org) and OSHA (https://www.osha.gov/safetypays/estimator) websites.

- Read the studies and reports cited in this chapter to learn more about where and how on-site PT saves money and adds value.

- Download the OSHA calculator and familiarize yourself with it.

- Create a spreadsheet to help you keep track of the injuries and illnesses you treat and prevent each month once you become an on-site PT.

- Choose a date each month—write it on your calendar—to issue a monthly report of your value to your client.

7

YOUR ON-SITE BUSINESS STRUCTURE

A huge part of your business model is deciding how to structure your on-site practice. As we've talked about, you can begin as an employee of a wellness company. If that's the case, you simply need to find a firm to hire you—no business structure needed. However, and as I've said several times in this book, to reap the real rewards of on-site practice requires you to be an independent contractor with your own business. Once you've committed to that, your next decision is how you want to start out.

- As a subcontractor?
- As a prime contractor?
- As a prime contractor with subcontractors or employees?
- As an owner of a traditional brick-and-mortar clinic with an on-site offering?

As you know, when I went out on my own, I didn't put any thought into the structure of my business. I didn't really know I had a choice. Once that new PT regulation went into effect in Colorado, it was either be unemployed or become a self-employed subcontractor to my previous employer. That subcontractor structure worked well for me at first—allowing me to stay at the placement where I'd been. However, over the years, as my competencies and confidence as an on-site PT and as a business owner grew, my business structure evolved to better serve my clients and patients, as well as increase my income and my independence.

Unlike me, you have the opportunity here to make a more conscious and considered decision about how you want your new business to operate. Each of the business structures discussed below has been proven successful for on-site PTs. None is particularly better than any other. Each has aspects for you to weigh.

The one that's right for you right now depends on your goals for your on-site practice, your confidence level in operating a business, and your intentions for your on-site practice and yourself. As you read about and evaluate each, think about which structure best suits your current resources, as well as the needs of the market in your area. Ask yourself which structure gives you the best start and the best foundation for building the career and life you envision.

STRUCTURE 1: SUBCONTRACTOR TO PRIME CONTRACTOR

Most physical therapists I know begin their on-site career as subcontractors by default. They fall into this structure (like I did). That's not necessarily a bad thing. Being a subcontractor allows you to experience how an on-site PT business operates without the responsibilities of managing clients, clinics, and patients on your own.

As a subcontractor, you contract through a prime contractor—typically a safety enterprise, health improvement firm, physical therapy or fitness business, or some type of health and wellness company. The prime contractor secures the clients—usually big, self-insured corporations or manufacturers with multiple locations. The prime then contracts with you and other subcontractors to staff their client's on-site clinics, provide services to their client's workforce, and fulfill their contractual obligations.

As a subcontractor, you are self-employed. You are not an employee. This means you are responsible for your own accounting, taxes, and any benefits you want to give yourself—like health insurance, sick days, or vacation days. You'll want to consult with an accountant and a lawyer (more details on that in Chapter 9) to ensure you're in compliance with all IRS obligations concerning subcontracting.

Being a subcontractor also means you can negotiate the terms of your contract with the prime contractor. For instance, as a subcontractor I negotiated a pay increase over what I made when I was an employee of the same company. Most contracts between primes and subs for on-site services include the scope of services (SOW), the number of hours per week you work, and an agreed-upon pay rate. (We get specific about contracts in Chapter 11.)

If you choose to start out as a subcontractor, consider looking for a prime contractor who does cater to large corporations. These bigger businesses usually have well-established on-site care, as well as mature safety cultures you can learn from. Also, these primes are likely to have more than one client, giving you the opportunity to experience different work environments and different types of injuries and safety situations—all of which will increase your knowledge and skill set. Best of all, bigger contractors with bigger clients tend to negotiate for multiyear contracts, giving you, as a sub, added stability in your income starting out.

For me, the biggest downside to being a subcontractor is losing direct communication with the client. All your requests, reporting, suggestions for improvements to the clinic and its programs, accolades, and quantified results must go through your prime, who then presents them (or not) to the client. The prime decides what gets discussed, acted on, or ignored—also, what, if anything, gets relayed back to you. With such a hurdle, information often moves slowly, to say the least.

Also, as a subcontractor, you don't have the autonomy you would as a prime (though you have more than you would as an employee). While your prime cannot legally supervise you or tell you "how" to do your job, they can decide which injury prevention platforms and reporting protocols you use. (Note that both you and your prime need to be careful here—too many regulations around "how" you do your job and the IRS may no longer consider you a subcontractor. To get clear on the difference between an "employee" and a "subcontractor," go to the "subcontractors' frequently asked questions" section at www.irs.gov. Also, before entering into a subcontract agreement, check with an attorney to ensure you and your prime contractor are in compliance with your status.)

The subcontractor structure for your on-site PT business might be the right structure for you to start out with if you are timid about being in business for yourself, need to learn more about on-site practice, or want to gain experience before going out on your own completely.

STRUCTURE 2: PRIME CONTRACTOR

If securing your own clients does not intimidate you and you feel confident in running a small business, you might look at structuring your business as prime contractor.

As a prime, you contract to provide your services directly with the client. There is no middleman. This gives you the potential to make more money than you would as a sub. Since you negotiate your contract one-to-one with the client, you also get to set the terms for how you work. You have full autonomy and full flexibility over how your practice operates—with the only restriction being that your client agrees.

To me, the greatest advantage of being a prime contractor is having control over my relationship with the client. As a prime, I have direct access. Whether I see a safety issue that needs attention or want to suggest an additional service, I can go straight to my client with my expertise and advice. As a prime, I'm able to give my clients my best, and that means my patients get my best as well.

For instance at one site, I started with a simple direct contract to provide prevention services ten hours per week. After one year, I saw that the client could benefit from having pre-employment testing and treatment on-site as well. I set up a meeting and provided them with the time and cost savings metrics that investing in these services through me would give them. They expanded my contract by twelve hours each week to include pre-employment testing and treatment.

When you directly contract with the client, you not only can suggest such changes but implement them quickly as well. You don't have to wait for some other entity to ruminate and negotiate. Remember, less bureaucracy equals more autonomy—and being a prime contractor gives you that.

The biggest downside—and once you get your business off the ground, it's not much of a downside—is finding and securing your own clients. (We take a deep dive into how to do this in Chapter 10.) The first client is the hardest to get. After that, my experience has been that as you grow your network and your reputation, signing clients becomes easier. If you do a good job for your current pt clients, within time, other businesses will hear about you and seek you out to brainstorm their business needs and to operate an on-site clinic for them.

By far, the biggest consideration when thinking about being a prime contractor is that every piece of managing the business is your responsibility. You write the proposal to get the business. You negotiate and write the contract to secure the business. (Again, proposals and contracts are coming up in Chapter 11). You are responsible for managing the day-to-day operations to meet the terms you've laid out for your client in that contract. When emergencies happen and mistakes get made—and both will—it's up to you and only you to remedy whatever goes wrong.

Because you are new to the on-site business and on your own, you may find your clients, at least at first, will be small, single-site, self-insured, local businesses and manufacturers. Be aware that these smaller enterprises aren't likely to have a well-developed safety culture. This can be an opportunity for you to be a leader for them and help them build one. But that also means you must stay current on safety culture, OSHA regulations, and workers' compensation laws. Remember, your client is looking to you to be the expert here.

One last thing—starting off as a prime contractor requires more of a financial investment up front than being a subcontractor. A prime needs more services from lawyers, accountants, and other professionals. You also need to invest more in marketing and networking for your sales effort.

So, structuring your business as a prime contractor works best for a PT who already has a network of potential clients, feels confident in their business skills, and understands the benefits of on-site care well enough to explain it (sell it) to potential clients. It also helps to be located in a market that has a good number of manufacturers who need on-site care, whether or not they know it.

STRUCTURE 2 A: PRIME CONTRACTOR WITH SUBCONTRACTORS OR EMPLOYEES

If you choose to be a prime contractor, it's not likely you'll be in need of subs or employees when you start out, but it's still worth having a good understanding of this structure for when you do need to hire to expand your business.

Under this structure, the big decision is whether your hires are going to be subcontractors or employees. Subcontractors are separate and distinct from your business—according to the IRS (and the IRS is who counts here.) This means that as the prime contractor, you cannot tell them specifically how to do their job or exactly how to schedule their work. Your only real control is to hire or fire them.

With employees, you have more of a say in what they do and how they do it. You can train employees, require them to do the job the way you want them to, make them use the tools you want them to, and even have them wear a uniform.

However, having employees comes with more management and fiscal responsibilities. For instance, your business must pay their withholding and employment-related taxes, as well as liability insurance and any benefits. (You'll want to check with your accountant here.)

When it came time for me to hire in my business, I decided that having employees rather than subcontractors was the right decision for me. I didn't want to trust the reputation of McCallum Physical Therapy to someone else's way of doing things. I train all my employees in my methodology, manage them closely, and regulate their actions on the job. By being able to oversee their work, I can be assured they are practicing the way I think is best for my clients and their workforce.

Whichever you as a prime contractor choose—employees or subcontractors—it's important that everyone involved is clear on the details of the employment relationship. Just as you would if you were a subcontractor, as a prime with any type of hires, you should consult an attorney to make sure you are in compliance with all IRS rules. You should also have a written contract between yourself and your hire that spells out the relationship.

Taking on hires allows you to have more clients, increase your income, and diversify your revenue streams. When the time comes, this is your structure for business expansion.

STRUCTURE 3: OFF-SITE CLINIC OFFERING ON-SITE SERVICES

If you are already an owner of an off-site or brick-and-mortar clinic, adding an on-site division can increase your profits without adding much to your overhead. This addition can be as simple as setting up a small clinic at a local employer to provide injury prevention consulting, as well as treatment.

Even better, this additional revenue stream is not dependent on insurance reimbursements or the volume of clinic visits. The payment is direct between the client and you. Of course, you'll want to have a system in place to see that you don't comingle funds with your brick-and-mortar clinic, as well as a system that prevents you from treating a patient both off-site and on.

If you do choose this structure, make sure your on-site staff understands that on-site care is different from the current clinic care model. Your on-site therapists will need to be educated in workplace care, injury prevention, safety culture, OSHA and workers' compensation laws and reporting. Expect a period of adjustment for both your PTs and your business.

(Beware that after working on-site, your PTs might not want to return to traditional practice.)

Clients in need of your on-site offerings will be small, local, self-insured businesses with high injury rates in material handling, distribution, transportation, or production industries. You might find them by checking which businesses are currently sending your brick-and-mortar clinic the most workers' compensation claims. If your workers' compensation contract allows, market your on-site service to these companies directly—with your cost savings and ROI (return on investment) of injury prevention infographic ready to go, of course.

For anyone who operates a brick-and-mortar clinic, adding on-site service is an easy, lucrative, and obvious avenue for growth.

COMBINING MODELS

Currently, my on-site PT business takes advantage of several of these structures. You should be prepared and flexible enough for your business to do the same in the future.

First, I am a subcontractor to a national health and wellness company that provides its clients with employee health improvement programs, including on-site medical clinics and PT programs. The client I'm subcontracted to has many plants across the United States. I oversee the on-site PT clinic in their Denver location. My contract with the prime is an annual contract—giving me and my business dependable monthly income.

Second—and here's the tricky part—because my subcontract with this prime is for fifty hours a week, my contract allows me to hire other PTs to provide services. So while I'm a subcontractor on this job, I'm also a subcontractor with employees.

And third, I do secure contracts directly with several clients on my own, making me a prime contractor with employees. As a prime, I negotiate my contract with either the company's head of safety or other human resources officers. Most of my contracts are annual and invoiced monthly—keeping the cash flow steady.

As my business proves, any of these business structures—or combination of structures—is likely to change as my business changes and other opportunities come my way. What I can say is through the upturns and downturns of the economy over the last decade or so, being able to be flexible with my business structure has worked to keep my businesses healthy and my personal economy in good shape.

EASING IN—INJURY PREVENTION SERVICES

If you're still feeling uneasy about the switch to on-site work, no matter what structure you choose to work under, consider aligning yourself with an injury prevention (IP)/industrial therapy company's particular methodology and utilizing their trainings to get started. When I first moved to on-site PT, I was an expert in movement, but I had no specific training with on-the-job injuries, job assessment, pre-employment testing, and the like. To boost my confidence and broaden my skills in these areas, I looked into training with an IP company. Not only did I find and take courses in the areas I knew I'd be dealing with as an on-site PT, but once I finished their training, I became a certified provider of their brand and methodology.

At first, this didn't mean much to my career. The wellness company I was employed by didn't use my certification to promote itself or me to clients. Still, I chose to pay the IP's licensing fee, so I would have access to their online ergonomic and document tools.

However, when I became a business owner seeking my own clients, my certification and affiliation with that IP company proved its worth. My licensing fee and yearly subscription to their training program automatically made me a provider in their network. I also stayed on their radar by staying active in their online community, contacting them about educational opportunities and keeping my skillset current through coursework in repetitive motion injuries, work-related injuries, basic orthopedic rehab, and more. When the IP company signed a national client with five job sites—one of which was in Colorado—they asked if I would be their PT subcontractor for that site. Though I already had several clients of my own, I decided to add their gig to my workload, which caused me to work fifty clinic hours a week for a while. However, once I had confidence that the contract would be ongoing, this became the push I needed to expand my own business. I hired my first employee to take over my hours at the IP's site. I trained them, and I oversaw (took responsibility for) their work.

Working through an IP company gave me some extra credibility and support as I started my business and then again when I was ready to grow. It can do the same for you. More than a few large IP companies provide training and certification in their approach to prevention and safety. As you investigate these companies, look for a philosophy or methodology that fits your own. Start with a Google search of "injury prevention companies," see what companies are out there (there are many), what courses they offer, which subcontract with PTs, and go from there.

NOW GET STARTED

As you'll learn soon enough for yourself, nothing in business is static. But then that's what makes running your own on-site PT practice continually interesting and rewarding. So don't be nervous. Don't overthink your structure. Simply choose the structure that looks like the best fit for you right now and get started. See how the structure works for you, for your clients or primes, and in your market.

If you find the structure isn't right, you can always change it. At the very least, always be prepared to modify your business structure to meet whatever opportunities come your way. As you grow in competency, the services you offer and how you offer them will evolve. As my own experience illustrates, the structure you start your on-site PT business with is not the structure you have forever. As to any trepidation you're feeling in this moment, opening and operating your own on-site practice will be the light at the end of the tunnel that keeps you moving forward and will give you a career and life you love.

EXERCISE:

Choosing a Structure

Questions

1. How would each type of business structure support or detract from your goals for becoming an on-site PT?

2. Are there state laws you need to consider as you choose a structure for your business?

3. What type of business structure appeals to you the most? Why?

4. What structure do you think is best to start your business with? Why?

5. What are the pros and cons for you of that structure?

6. Do you see your business growing into a different structure eventually? If so, how can you build your business now to support that growth later? (This is not something you need to know immediately but something you should keep in the back of your head as you move forward.)

Activities

- Read through each structure slowly. Weigh the pros and cons. Choose the one that looks like the best fit for you now.

- If aligning with an IP company seems like a good route for you, start researching. Look into the various companies out there, the methodologies they offer, and how they work.

8

—

ON-SITE PT AS ENTREPRENEUR

When I committed to making the move from employee to entrepreneur, I could not imagine myself as a business owner. However, by the time I was running my own business, I realized nothing about it was as difficult or mysterious as I'd made it out to be. I mean, I had to get a small business attorney, learn how to read a contract, figure out how much money I needed (wanted) to make, and learn how to do small business accounting (QuickBooks is a life saver). But all that stuff, the stuff I was scared of—the business stuff—was relatively easy to both figure out and do.

It turns out the biggest obstacle to making a smooth transition from employee to entrepreneur is in our heads. It's our mindset—in other words, our beliefs about what being entrepreneurs means and what it looks like. FYI, most of us have it wrong.

Instead of worrying about what I didn't know about business (I now know there will always be something I don't know), my focus should have been on what would be required of me personally and professionally as a business owner and making sure those things were in place. I didn't know that then. Luckily, you will now. To ease your concerns and give you confidence in your abilities to own and operate an on-site PT business, this last component in your business plan is to define and continue to develop your entrepreneurial mindset.

BUT THE RISKS . . .

Let's start by addressing "risk." The minute you tell someone you're going to quit your job and open your own business, they're likely to feel the need to point out that working for yourself is "risky." They might even back up their worry with the worn-out statistic that 50 percent of small businesses fail within the first five years.

For me, operating my own on-site PT service for the last decade has proven more secure and steady than working in a brick-and-mortar clinic. My successes are tied directly to my work results, not some unachievable clinic metric or complicated bonus structure. If there's a reduction in the business's income, I'm not going to lay myself off or cut my hours back. As the owner, I have the agency to get more clients, raise my rates, increase my services to existing clients, whatever it takes to get the cash flowing again. The bottom line is, as an entrepreneur, I have more control over my employment status, my income, and my life—not less.

If you feel a little scared about becoming a business owner, that's natural. Feeling apprehension is a normal part of starting something new, anything new. In general, it's the uncertainty of a novel situation that makes us feel nervous—not the situation itself. So yes, from where you sit now, the thought of entrepreneurship may be a little unsettling. But it should also feel exciting and empowering—because it is.

YOU AS ENTREPRENEUR

The biggest difference between being an employee and being an entrepreneur is the level and scope of your responsibilities. As an employee, you take responsibility for the quality of care you deliver to your patients. You might also feel obligated to be a good team player for coworkers and to do your best for your clinic. But as an employee, your responsibilities and your work end at the clinic door. Once you leave for the day, you aren't thinking about how to make the business more efficient, what new services might help your employer reach their business goals, or how to make the patient experience better. (If you are, you likely already have an entrepreneurial mindset.)

As a business owner, however, when you're not working with patients, you're running your business and thinking about all those things. Whether you do the work yourself or contract it out, every aspect of the business is your responsibility—the quality of care, the range of care, the marketing, sales, administration, profitability, etc. All final decisions become yours. Not everyone is cut out for this. It takes a certain kind of person to embrace this level of responsibility and see the independence as a reward in itself.

Before I opened my business, I thought entrepreneurs were visionaries with endless ideas, front-of-the-curve type of people, charismatic leaders, and smooth talkers. I was none of those things. But when I looked up the term "entrepreneur" in *Merriam Webster*, I found the definition was much more straightforward than all that. According to the dictionary, an entrepreneur is "one who organizes, manages, and assumes the risks of a business enterprise." I knew that was someone I could be. The organizing and managing I already had down. The risk-taking I could teach myself to get used to. Taking my research a little further—reading several books on entrepreneurship and speaking with friends who were business owners—I found five traits to be essential to the entrepreneurial mindset:

1. You must be mature.

Being mature means being able to think calmly and rationally no matter how crazy the world or the people around you are. A mature person is not reactive. You don't take things personally. Your emotions don't make your decisions. You know your values, you know your goals for yourself and your business, and you make your decisions guided by them.

As a mature person, you take responsibility for your actions and decisions. You don't feel the need to blame others. You don't waste time on excuses. You accept reality and make your next move based on it. When a decision doesn't produce the outcome you want, you change course without consulting your ego. When you make a mistake, you own it, apologize, and correct it.

2. You must be a self-starter.

When you're the boss, there's no one to tell you what to do or what needs to be done. So to run your own business, you must be the kind of person who works well on their own without direction. You must be unafraid to solve problems, think on your feet, and make a decision when one is needed (and those decisions will be needed more than you can imagine right now.)

3. You must be secure enough to handle risk and rejection.

So much in business comes down to the ask. And so many people are afraid of asking because they're afraid of the word "no." They're afraid of rejection.

As an entrepreneur, asking is something you do multiple times a day, every day. Asking is how you get clients, how you get a fair deal, how problems get solved, and how you learn things. You can't afford not to ask. Asking is how business gets done. So getting turned down now and then is part of the job.

This doesn't mean you have to love rejection. Everybody would rather hear "yes" than "no." But you can't run a business if your fear of rejection prevents you from asking for what you need. You have to accept "no" for what it is (and no more), dust yourself off, and come up with another way to get what you were asking for. That's the only way to reach your goals and advance your business.

Years ago in a marketing workshop, I learned that "no" isn't a hard stop or a reflection of me as a person. "No" is simply a pause on the way to "yes." It's an invitation to reevaluate your ask and make the offer more beneficial for both parties.

Be honest with yourself here. If "no" is a hard stop for you, if you find the thought of rejection paralyzing, self-employment may not be the best career choice for you. If, however, you can see "no" as a new piece of information, a tool for learning, and a step toward "yes," then you are well on your way to the mindset needed to be responsible for a business.

Don't sell yourself short. When I started out, I thought of myself as someone who avoided rejection at all costs. But when I looked a little more deeply, I realized I often heard "no" from patients when prescribing treatment or time off or something else they didn't want to hear. Their "nos" never stopped me. I always figured out another way to reach them and get them the care they needed. I realized these were skills and a mindset I was already employing and could now translate to my business.

As long as we're on the subject of rejection, as a business owner, you also must be able to reject things and people who don't serve your business well. You must be okay with firing employees and vendors who aren't working out, turning down opportunities that aren't right for your business, and sometimes even letting clients go to make room for clients that are a better fit.

Getting comfortable with rejection (both the being and the doing) is a muscle. When you put conviction and thoughtfulness behind it, it does get easier, though it never fully becomes enjoyable—which is probably a good thing.

4. You must be organized and dependable.

Believe it or not, this is where so many stereotypical "entrepreneurial types" fall short. Being successful in business isn't only about starting something—you must also be able to follow through. This is especially true when your business is being responsible for other people's health.

Your clients and your patients depend on you to open your on-site clinic on time (or make sure someone does). They expect you to be up-to-date on the latest and best practices in your field, to help them stay well and uninjured, and to keep meticulous records of it all.

Your business needs you to be meticulous too. Being organized is, of course, about proper bookkeeping, making sure all licensure is up to date, and all the paperwork is filed. But it's also about scheduling, tracking sales calls, updating contracts, replying to emails, staying on top of the laws that govern your practice, and taking care of the hundreds of other details that make your business run.

While you can and should hire out some of this work, you are the one who is ultimately responsible for seeing everything gets done. Being organized and dependable is nonnegotiable for an entrepreneur.

5. You must be a leader—in your own way.

Just as I never thought of myself as an entrepreneur before I opened my own business, I never thought of myself as a leader. But to own a business is to lead. Your clients, your patients, your employees (if you have any), and your professional team (lawyers, accountants, etc.) all look to you for direction.

As a licensed, working PT, you're already a leader in many ways. Every day, you take charge of your patients and their care. Also, in taking the initiative to look into opening your own on-site PT service, you're showing leadership right now over your career and life.

I used to think leaders had to be out-in-front kind of people. I've since learned there are all types. I like to think I'm the kind who leads by example. As you begin to think of yourself as a business owner and do the work to open your business, you'll notice yourself becoming a leader in your own way with your own style.

Not every PT (or person) has an entrepreneurial mindset or the inclination to have their own business. But because of our PT training and our natural disposition toward taking charge, preempting problems, and detailed thoroughness, more of us have what it takes to be business owners than you might think.

DOTTING YOUR "I's"

To support your mindset—and your business—as you begin to execute your business plan, make sure you have your credentials and licensing in order and use your required continuing education to gain more knowledge pertinent to operating an on-site clinic.

For credentials, you want to at least have a master's degree in physical therapy from an accredited PT school. A doctor of physical therapy (DPT), of course, is even better. I'd already started my on-site business when I went back to school to get my doctorate in physical therapy. In addition to increasing my knowledge and skills, being in school upped my game in terms of networking, critical thinking, and confidence in taking risks.

Naturally, you want to be sure you're licensed to practice in the state where you're going to open your business. If your plan includes virtual PT for employees in other states, look into PT compact licensure (https:// ptcompact.org)—which some states allow. Also, as noted in Chapter 4, be sure to review and maintain a thorough understanding of the direct-access laws in your state.

As you get closer to opening your business, be sure any continuing education deepens the knowledge and skills you'll need for on-site practice. For instance, sign up for professional courses in ergonomics, material handling, OSHA first aid, diversity training, and infection control. Think about injuries and issues your clients' workforces are likely to present with and search for training that targets them. While there is no shortage of paid courses in continuing education, some free resources for useful classes for on-site care include:

- Musculoskeletal Disorders (MSD)
  https://www.osha.gov/ergonomics
  https://www.cdc.gov/workplacehealthpromotion/index.html

- Injury Prevention
  https://www.osha.gov/safety-management/hazard-prevention

- Ergonomics and Workflow
  https://www.cdc.gov/niosh/topics/ergonomics/default.html
  https://www.cdc.gov/niosh/topics/PTD/

- Job Demands Analysis
  https://www.bls.gov/ors/factsheet/physical-072015.htm

- Pre-Employment Testing
  https://www.eeoc.gov/laws/guidance/employment-tests-and-selection-procedures

- Workplace First Aid
  https://www.osha.gov/medical-first-aid

GET SUPPORT FOR THE BUSINESS STUFF

Part of the entrepreneurial mindset is knowing when to get help and cultivating competent and reliable sources to give it to you. As soon as I committed to starting my own business, I reached out to my connections in PT clinics and other small businesses. I let them know my plans, my fears, and my business goals. I asked for any help or advice they wanted to give. No tip was too small—from how to do payroll taxes to interviewing to community resources that would help me. In those moments of self-doubt ("Can I really do this?"), I found my courage through small moments of independent learning and large moments of reassurance from others.

Being self-employed does not mean going it alone. You need a community of other business owners to fill in the gaps of your knowledge and to let you know they've been where you are and everything will be all right. Other small business owners—especially other on-site PTs—want you to succeed and will go out of their way to share their experiences and support you.

To build such a community, make a list of everyone you know who knows something different than you and contact them. I spoke with old clients, a retired tax preparer, other PTs, and a small business lawyer who was a friend of a friend. Also pull into your group nonprofits whose mission is to help people just like you navigate the ins and outs of operating a small business. Several networking and learning groups I used included:

- Small Business Association
- LinkedIn
- Small Business Development Center
- SCORE Business Mentoring
- WBENC (Women's Business Enterprise National Council)

Beyond gaining the benefits of their expertise, I found most of these groups cross-promoted within their membership. There is no need to re-invent the wheel here. Everything you need to know about starting a successful on-site PT business, operating one, and growing one has been done by someone else. Therefore, it can be learned by connecting to the right people and organizations.

MAKING THE SHIFT: FROM EMPLOYEE TO ENTREPRENEUR

From the moment you put your business plan into action, you will be a business owner, an entrepreneur, the principal of your operation. For most of us PTs, that's a significant shift in the way we think about work, about our practice, and about ourselves.

But here's the thing: Like me, you already know how to provide PT services. And you know you can (and will) learn the business parts. You also know you are going to make mistakes as you grow your business, likely sell yourself short sometimes, and live through ups and downs. Having a strong entrepreneurial mindset—not an MBA—is what will carry you through it all.

I can also tell you that many physical therapists have been where you are right now and today are running successful on-site PT businesses, glad they made the shift, and fully confident that they wouldn't return to being an employee if they could. That includes me. Soon it will include you too.

EXERCISE:
Creating a Business State of Mind

Questions

1. What fears do you have about being a business owner?
2. Are there any fears that can't be overcome with information and practice?
3. Do you possess the qualities discussed in this chapter that are necessary to be an entrepreneur? Any you might need to work on?
4. Do you have the credentials needed to become an on-site PT?

Activities

- Ensure you are current with state laws on compact licensure (https://ptcompact.org) and direct access (https://www.apta.org/advocacy/issues/direct-access-advocacy/direct-access-by-state).
- Create a clear-cut response for people who tell you that opening your own business is too risky and you should keep the job you have.
- Sign up for continuing education classes in subjects that can advance your on-site work.
- Make a plan to network with other small business owners and small business groups to get your questions answered and your fears calmed.

Section Three

OPENING AND OPERATING YOUR ON-SITE PRACTICE

In this last section, we get into the details of running your on-site PT business. Here you'll learn exactly what you need—lists and charts included—to get your practice open, get your first client, and get to work.

9

———

YOUR BASE OF SUPPORT: PUTTING YOUR TEAM TOGETHER

When it comes to PT, you are the expert. But when it comes to setting up and operating a fully legal, properly documented, and well-protected business, you probably aren't quite sure what you need to know, let alone how to make it happen. The good news here is you don't have to know. You can and should hire those things out.

Ensuring a smooth operation means getting advice and services from a team of professionals who know what your business needs. Before opening your on-site practice, you should secure an attorney, an accountant, and an insurance agent. As your business grows, you might also want to look into hiring a virtual assistant, a payroll vendor, and any other professional who can shorten your learning curve and help you to make your business all you want it to be.

YOUR ATTORNEY

When I opened McCallum Physical Therapy, I didn't know any business attorneys or what exactly I would use one for. On the advice of my local Small

Business Association (SBA) mentor (a service available to you, too, through your local SBA), I did some research about legal considerations for small businesses. I started with the SBA website (SBA.gov). I also talked with the Colorado-based lobbyist for the APTA. And I asked for advice and recommendations from some PTs I knew who ran their own clinics, as well as friends who were small-business owners.

From those conversations, I gained a general idea of what legal services my business might need. I also secured the names of three attorneys to look into. The first one I interviewed practiced at a firm that specialized in large PT clinics, other types of rehab centers, and franchise markets. He charged a minimum of $500 per consultation. Needless to say, he wasn't the right fit for my one-person start-up or my budget.

The second was a friend of a PT colleague. Though he knew his stuff, had a background with small business, and was very generous about answering my questions, I never felt we connected or that he fully understood my vision for my business. By the way, "not feeling a connection" is a perfectly valid reason for not hiring a professional. You want to be completely comfortable and be able to talk freely with the people you're paying to help you. There was nothing wrong with him; he seemed like a great guy. It just wasn't a match.

The third attorney—who was recommended by my SBA mentor—was in practice for herself. As a small-business owner, she understood my challenges firsthand. In my free fifteen-minute consultation with her—which she offered to confirm her skill set met my needs (something I really appreciated)—I learned that she had a good deal of experience setting up small PT businesses like mine and she specialized in contracts, an area I knew would be critical to my success. Also, she billed by the tenth of an hour (every six minutes). I would only pay for the time I used. Her experience and the way she worked were right in line with my needs and my budget. No surprise, I chose her to help get me started.

Because of the research I'd done, I had an idea of what I needed her help with. But I had no idea how valuable her legal expertise would be for my business. Here are just a few of the areas where her counsel proved invaluable—areas you might want to explore with your own attorney. (Just a note here: In no way is anything written in this section or in this book to be taken as legal advice. I am not a lawyer. Any legal advice you use should come from a licensed, practicing attorney—which is the point of this chapter, after all.)

Setting up your business as its own entity

Many small business owners operate as sole proprietors, which is the easiest type of business to initiate, no paperwork involved. However, as a sole proprietor, you and your business are one and the same in the eyes of the IRS and the law—meaning your business profit is your personal profit and your business liabilities are your personal liabilities. That can be risky, especially when your business is in health care.

Incorporating your business separates you and your business into two different entities—which can offer tax benefits, but more importantly, limits your business liability to your business assets. There are four basic types of legal business structures—limited liability corporations (LLCs), partnerships, S Corps, and C Corps. While you can and should find details on each of these structures at irs.gov, selecting which is right for your business is something to discuss with an attorney. You want to have a full understanding of the ins and outs of each type for your particular situation.

Small businesses like on-site practices are typically LLCs or S Corps. Many entrepreneurs choose an LLC structure because it's easy to set up and still provides personal liability protection. However, after talking with my lawyer and CPA, I decided on the S Corp. While an S Corp takes more effort (and a little more cost) to establish and maintain, it does provide a more defined separation between my business and my personal assets, along with a tax structure that suits me better.

Once you decide on how you want to incorporate, your attorney can then file the necessary paperwork with the state. If you wish, you can also hire your attorney to file your annual corporation review with the state. I do. Filing this review isn't difficult, but handing it over to my attorney means one less thing on my to-do list. It also keeps her current with changes in my business.

Writing articles of incorporation and bylaws

If you choose to be an S Corp, like me, then filing with the state means having articles of incorporation and bylaws, and at least one shareholder. All things an attorney can explain and help you secure. While bylaws and articles of incorporation are technical, dry documents, they are wonderful at guiding and protecting your business when there is a dispute or something goes wrong.

Of course, my lawyer knew what needed to be included in each and wrote them up for me, consulting with me all along the way. She also counseled me on the details of having at least one shareholder for the S Corp, as well as what both my shareholder and my legal responsibilities and duties were to the corporation (e.g., holding an annual "stockholder" meeting). We structured my S Corp with me as the sole shareholder. So, I'm the only person financially vested in the company.

Ensuring adherence to the requirements of the state physical therapy board

Every state PT board has its own rules and regulations when it comes to PT practices. The Colorado Physical Therapy Board, for example, requires that any incorporated practice must have the words "professional company," "professional corporation," or the abbreviation "PC" after their name. So once I incorporated, McCallum Physical Therapy needed to become McCallum Physical Therapy PC on all formal documents, as well as my business card, stationery, etc.

My attorney informed me of this. It wasn't something I even knew I needed to know—just one of many, many important details in opening a business that I would have missed without professional assistance.

File for a city business license

While this typically isn't a difficult thing to do, allowing your attorney to do it gives you the added protection of knowing this all-important document was filled out properly and filed correctly with your city.

Contract review

Contracts are how we operate as on-site PTs. They spell out the terms of our work with our clients. Good ones make sure everyone is clear on expectations, and that keeps your clients happy. Should something go wrong—and sometimes things go wrong—contracts give everyone a neutral document to look at to settle the dispute.

Whether I am renewing a contract with the same language, signing a contract with a new client, or subcontracting with a prime for a client, I have my attorney review the contract. She not only answers all my questions and makes sure I understand what I am agreeing to, but she also verifies the contract is fair and accurate.

Advising on employee law

The area of personnel management is legally complicated, to say the least. Job listings, interviewing, hiring, and terminating are minefields for legal mistakes that can get you sued and hurt your reputation. In addition to having my lawyer educate me about employee law, I also have her review all communications with anyone I hire—from job listings to emails to contracts.

This is far from an exhaustive list of the services your attorney can and will provide for your business. I have used my lawyer's services not only for situations in a purely legal context but also for those that require business acumen and delicate steps. For instance, a situation where growing my business might have the appearance of a conflict of interest or direct competition with my current client. Of course, I don't want to anger my current client by "bypassing" their process or seeming disloyal. My attorney can both reassure me that I am adhering to my contract with my client, while advising me on how to present my "growth" in such a way that my client doesn't feel I've sidestepped them or their process.

When you run a business, there are unknowns at every corner. Not to mention, the law changes. A good attorney who knows both you and your business is an invaluable resource. I've been with my attorney for more than a decade now. She is someone I never hesitate to turn to, and her expertise is something I never hesitate to use.

YOUR ACCOUNTANT/TAX PREPARER

I found my certified public accountant (CPA) through my lawyer, which isn't unusual in the world of small business. As you'll soon find out, small-business owners tend to support one another. When we find someone we like working with and who does their job well, we refer them, and in return, they refer us. When it comes to hiring your own CPA—if you're not so lucky as to have a recommendation fall in your lap, then ask around, just as you did when you were looking for a lawyer.

The primary reason to hire a CPA is taxes. Especially when you incorporate, your taxes become more complicated. (You can say goodbye to the 1040EZ tax form.) Also, tax laws change every year. Business tax laws even more so. Taxes are also the reason to choose a CPA over a regular accountant. The CPA after their name tells you they've passed a rigorous exam, participate in continuing education to maintain their certification, and know the current tax code inside out.

In addition to tax preparation, my CPA provided me with smart, specific-to-me fiscal advice right from the start. For instance, when I was choosing between becoming an LLC vs. an S Corp, he was able to calculate that I—in my situation—would pay less in personal tax as an S Corp than an LLC. When I mentioned that I needed some start-up funding, he suggested that I personally loan my S Corp money, so I wouldn't need to go to a bank and pay them interest on start-up funds. He also made sure I documented the loan correctly, paid myself back correctly, and completed the promissory note correctly. Perhaps most importantly, my CPA insisted from the start that I pay myself a salary. And because I was an S Corp, he also told me to make a regular shareholder distribution to myself to maximize my take-home pay based on tax laws. I never would have known to do any of this or how to do it on my own.

Let me stress here, no matter what type of business or corporation you decide on, you should ask your accountant about making provisions to pay yourself a salary. Every financial advisor I talk to has said that one of the biggest mistakes small business owners make is not paying themselves a regular amount as soon as possible in their endeavor. Work with your accountant to make this happen for you.

I do not use my CPA's firm for daily bookkeeping. For most small businesses, hiring out bookkeeping isn't necessary. For on-site PT practices, our billing is usually limited to just a few clients and our expenses are not difficult to track. A popular accounting software program serves my needs well and provides my CPA with all the reports and information he needs.

There are many good accounting software programs out there. Again, ask around to see what people use. Whichever you choose, I recommend taking the free course that most of them offer to become efficient using it. I did not do this at first and struggled.

YOUR INSURANCE AGENT

Finding the right insurance agent can prove more difficult than finding a CPA or lawyer because on-site PT businesses need some industry-specific insurance. When I was first looking, I turned to the internet and searched terms such as "workers' compensation" and "commercial insurance." I filled out a ton of online forms at various insurance sites.

What I discovered was that many agents and brokers had only a few products to sell when it came to business insurance and would do everything they could to convince me that their products worked for my business. They did not. Pretty quickly, I saw I needed an agent who was willing to take the time to understand my business, truly advise me, and put together an insurance package that would keep my on-site PT practice safe. I ended up finding just such an agent on the state workers' compensation website.

When you find yours, here are some policy areas to be sure to ask about and explore:

Professional liability and malpractice insurance

As employees, most PTs carry this type of insurance. However, as a business owner, you likely need to upgrade your professional liability and malpractice insurance to cover your increased assets and exposure. My current policy, for instance, is based on the number of employees I have. Also, be aware that often your clients will have their own requirements as to the level of liability and malpractice insurance you must carry. This is something you want to discuss with your agent to make sure your policy has the flexibility to meet varying needs.

Commercial automobile insurance

Now that you're in business, you want to be sure your auto insurance covers your car for both personal and business use. As with your regular automobile policy, you can choose to include medical payments, un-/under-insured drivers, rental car, roadside service, etc. Again, this is where the advice of a good agent can help so much.

Business owner's insurance (sometimes called commercial general liability)

This policy protects your business from property damage, identity theft, a data breach, and general liability. Ask your agent to advise you on what to include in this policy and how much to insure your business for. Obviously, as the business grows and becomes more valuable, this policy should grow and the coverage increase as well.

Workers' compensation insurance

If you have employees, your business must carry this insurance. The rate is based on your industry, how many employees you have, and your annual payroll. To save money, I opted to leave myself off my workers' compensation policy. If anything happens to me, my plan is to use my personal health insurance. Again, your agent can walk you through the ins and outs of this mandated insurance.

Personal health insurance

In the United States, health insurance presents a challenge for many small business owners—those of us who own on-site PT businesses are no exception. An agent can be crucial here in helping you understand your options. For now, you yourself need coverage. In the future, you may need to consider whether it's feasible to cover employees. (I do not offer a stipend or health insurance to my employees. My small company size and the part-time status of my employees makes me exempt from the Affordable Care Act mandate.)

Depending on your income, personal health insurance from the Affordable Care Act marketplace can be affordable if you qualify for a subsidy. It can be expensive if you don't. Whatever your situation, it's worth the effort to look into it (health care.gov) and discuss it with a knowledgeable agent.

All the types of insurance I mentioned above can be essential to your business, but how you package the policies is up to you and your insurance agent. Remember, your clients may have specific coverage amounts that they require all vendors to carry and may also want to be included on the certificate of insurance. This will be a nonnegotiable portion of your contract with them. So be prepared. Understand that insurance is and likely always will be a major cost for your business. (To give you an idea, my total insurance expenditure for my first year in business was a little more than $8,000.) Consequently, when it comes to insurance, you want to shop around.

OTHER PROFESSIONALS TO CONSIDER

As your business grows, it's likely your team will need to grow as well. Here are some team members (and technologies) to consider:

Virtual assistants

Many entrepreneurs I know use virtual assistants (VAs). VAs, for the most part, take care of administrative tasks you no longer have time for or you simply don't want to do any longer. Because they are contract workers, you can hire them as needed for a single project or on an ongoing basis for only the hours you need each week.

Work-saving technologies

Personally, I haven't hired a VA, because technology has rescued me from becoming buried in administrative tasks as business has increased. For instance, electronic medical records (EMRs) handle most of my clinic work. They take care of all my scheduling needs and send appointment reminders automatically.

To keep track of clients, my prospects, and other contacts, I've invested in customer relationship management (CRM) software. Essentially, CRMs do everything from organizing your contacts to managing sales leads to sending texts and emails automatically. CRMs also produce data that can help you identify areas of growth in your business—for instance, where your best client opportunities are. I think of my CMR as an address book with superpowers.

Most CMRs offer limited free services. This is a great way to try out different ones and see which fits your business best. Then when you need to, you can opt into the paid services, such as marketing, contact verifications, and lead generation.

Payroll vendor

One professional I did add to my team as my business grew was a payroll vendor. A payroll vendor handles all the details of payroll—federal and state taxes, Medicare and social security withholding, unemployment taxes and filing, quarterly filings, etc. When it came to my employees, I didn't want to assume the risk associated with making payroll errors. Also, since my employees don't work in one location, a payroll agency could get them their paycheck faster than I could.

This didn't negate my educating myself about those payroll details, however. Understanding what a well-run payroll is let me know what to look for when choosing a vendor and how to judge the quality of their work once I hired them.

In addition to the "other professionals" listed here, know that you'll use some professionals intermittently, on an as-needed basis. Over the years, I have hired various marketing professionals as needed. I had a business advisor for a few years, and every year, I hire an educator to review HIPAA, CPR, etc., with my employees.

GO TEAM!

As you'll discover, there are professionals out there to meet just about any business need you might have. Once your business gets going, your time is better invested in doing things you can't hire out.

Having an attorney, an accountant, and an insurance agent on your team is standard and necessary. When it comes to hiring other professional services—such as public relations services, IT services, project management—think about where your talents lie and where they don't, what you like to do and what you don't, and think about where your lack of expertise in the area might cost your business more than investing in professional help.

Pricing, of course, varies for everything. Do not hesitate to get a quote and then call around for other quotes. Always ask friends and colleagues for referrals (but don't hire friends and family; it typically doesn't turn out well.) Try people out. Make your needs known. Remember, these professionals work for you. It's your team, after all. If you aren't satisfied, find another vendor—there are plenty of them out there in every category.

To operate a well-run business, you don't have to know everything about everything. Behind every great business is a great team—even if technically, you are a solo-preneur.

....

EXERCISE:
Your Team

....

Questions

1. Have you ever worked with a team of professionals before? What concerns do you have about having a team?

2. If you currently have a lawyer, accountant, and insurance agent, would they be appropriate to help you open and manage your on-site practice? If not, can they give you guidance toward someone in their field who could?

Activities

- Look into securing a Small Business Association mentor to help you through this team-building process (www.score.org).

- Make a list of anyone else you can reach out to in your community to get recommendations for the professionals you need.

- Create a questionnaire for each type of professional you are going to interview.

- If you think you are going to hire any professionals beyond attorneys, accountants, and insurance agents, create detailed job descriptions for them before you search for them.

10

WHERE CLIENTS COME FROM —MARKETING

Whenever I talk with PTs about starting an on-site practice, they show the most resistance to marketing their business. At the mention of the "m" word, many say things like: "I don't think I'd be good at marketing." "I don't know the first thing about sales." "I just don't have what it takes to get clients."

Marketing is something I struggled with at first too. I thought marketing would require me to be an aggressive salesperson. I thought I'd have to be extroverted, convincing, pushy, and not 100 percent looking out for my clients' best interests. I knew that just wasn't (and isn't) me.

If those are your thoughts, I want you to know:

- You're already good at marketing, and I'll prove that to you.
- Effective marketing and selling are not about being pushy and selfish, just the opposite.
- Marketing your business well and securing clients (the sale) isn't a personality contest.

Marketing is something that, in my experience, we PTs do naturally.

YOU'VE ALWAYS BEEN IN MARKETING

Marketing is making potential clients aware that you understand their problem and can solve it (with your services). Sales is turning those prospects into paying clients. Being successful at marketing and sales is nothing more than connecting, educating, serving, and then monitoring to identify further needs.

Those are things PTs do every day in the clinic—things we're good at. Every appointment you have begins with connecting to your patients by listening to their problems and taking their history. You then educate them as to how specifically PT (the service you offer) can help improve or fix whatever is wrong and get them to their goal of restoring their health. You share with them your knowledge of and belief in a healthy lifestyle, active rehab, and the power of the body and mind to heal. You inform them as to how it works. Based on the information you've shared, they "buy in." That's marketing.

Once they agree to a treatment you've presented (i.e., you make a sale!), you serve them—building trust and your relationship by delivering a high-quality experience with promised outcomes. Also, you continue to monitor your patients—ensuring whatever brought them to you is resolved and looking for any other issues you can help with (i.e., new sales opportunities). That's advanced marketing—and as a PT you do it every day.

As a clinician, I always felt confident in my skills "selling" patients on themselves, the benefits of PT, and their recovery. As a new business owner, I realized all I needed to do was to transfer that confidence and skill to helping potential clients understand the benefits to their company of working with my company. In the end, marketing is finding out what your clients need and ensuring they get it. No aggressive tactics, no pushiness needed.

TARGET YOUR MARKET

As a small business owner, your resources are limited. So you only want to invest your marketing energy and dollars connecting with companies that are the right fit for you—and vice versa. Each self-insured company has its own set of challenges, needs, and expectations. Your business too has needs, expectations, and a protocol for how you want to work. Your ideal clients are companies where you can do your best work; those who would benefit most from your services. To define and identify them, look at three factors: your location, the structure of your business, and the scope of your services.

Since physical therapy is an in-person service, your clients need to be in your area—at least for now, when you are "the staff" at the clinic site. Decide what commute length is acceptable, get out a map, and draw a circle in that mileage radius. That's your market area. (As your business grows and you hire employees or subcontractors, you may choose to become a regional or national business. But for now, you're a local business.)

Whether you've structured your business as a prime contractor or a subcontractor, you begin with an online search for self-insured companies in manufacturing, distribution, transportation, construction, and other industries that have jobs with moderate to heavy physical demands. Also look for companies in this category that have retention issues; as we discussed, presenteeism and absenteeism are as big of a problem for employers as injury.

To develop my first prospect list, I searched for "self-insured companies in Colorado" and found several near me. I then narrowed my search to "medical claims for self-insured companies in Colorado." With that, I landed on the state's workers' compensation site, which had a list of all self-insured companies in the state. So you might want to check to see if your state's workers' compensation site has a similar list. If it does, also check out the most common injuries in each of your local industries—and be sure your services address them.

Another productive online search option is the "safety" route. Working through ZoomInfo, Limeleads, or other database companies, search for names of safety managers at companies in your market area. Note the companies they work for. Be aware that some companies have "publicity restricted" clauses and don't allow their vendors to promote them as a customer. But others are happy to be noted—so if you check out the "satisfied customer" or "testimonials" section, you're likely to get some leads. Once you have a few names, pull up your state's Department of Labor's information data to research the customer company's workers' compensation claims.

This combination of information can give you an idea of which companies might have on-site services. At the very least, it will give you a starting point when you make a call to their risk manager, safety representative, or occupational health manager. In addition, you can learn who works directly with local providers and who contracts with large wellness or rehabilitation firms to staff their on-site clinics. All great insights to help you decide who might be a good prospect.

As you do this research, make a spreadsheet of your findings with the company name, the safety manager's name, contact information, and the details you uncovered. You want this information at your fingertips.

Don't overlook your current place of employment as a resource for identifying ideal clients. Whether you own a brick-and-mortar PT clinic or work at one, start paying attention to where your patients come from. Are they making a workers' compensation claim? Are their companies self-insured? Do those companies have a wellness program? Ask. How many other patients a month are you treating from that same company? Look it up. Ask your patients who to talk to at their company and for an introduction, if they're willing. Add your findings to your spreadsheet.

If your business is structured as a prime contracting company, you should have what you need here for a decent prospect list. If you're looking to be a subcontractor, you need to do all the above and find out which of the major prime contractors serve your area. Search the web for "corporate health and wellness companies" or "corporate wellness providers." Try human resource–specific sites, such as the Society for Human Resource Management. Organizations like these often recommend (and rate) vendors. Also, check out research organization databases such as Rand, Kaiser Family Foundation, and Accenture. Then match these prime contractors to the companies in your area.

RESEARCH BEFORE REACHING OUT

Now that you have a prospect list, learn all you can about each company before approaching them. Remember, you're working to establish a relationship that lasts and grows, adding more value to their business and yours. Whether you're approaching a company directly or approaching a prime as a subcontractor, you want to be seen as an asset from the start. That means going in knowing who your client is, what they might need (but don't assume, always listen), and what questions to ask them. Primarily, you want to know if they're the kind of operation you'd like to work for.

Company websites can give you a feel for this. Look at their history. Look into what they do and how they do it. Look for their mission, their vision, and their values. Is this a company you respect, who respects its employees, and who you think will respect you? See if you can find a copy of the annual report online. Inside it is a wealth of information from organizational charts to contact information.

To get beyond the company's own marketing copy, look for online reviews. What do customers and employees say? In addition to Google and Yahoo, look at Glassdoor—where employees post about their experiences. If you see complaints related to injuries, not feeling cared for, or employee retention, make a note. These may be areas where they need your help.

For companies with on-site clinics, find out if they have PT on-site. If you can't find this information online, pick up the phone. I've called many a company's general number and asked the operator about the company's benefits. It took a little nerve, but I got the information I needed.

If you're researching prime contractors, look to their website to confirm they do business in your area and see what services they offer. What is their business philosophy? How are they structured? Are they looking for subcontractors? What are their hiring practices? Go to reviews to find out what their reputation is among their clients and subcontractors.

Many companies promote their procurement efforts in "supplier diversity." If you are a minority/women-owned/certified small business, there may be extra incentive for the potential prime or client to look at your services, as it helps them meet their diversity goals. While this would never be the primary reason they'd choose your company, it can be a good foot-in-the-door relationship starter.

Once you have a general idea of who these client-companies and/or prime contractors are, focus your research on where you and your business can add value to theirs. When you meet with them, you want to present your services as an investment with a clear return. So, before your meeting, find the answers to these questions:

- Do they or the companies they contract with have high rehab costs due to insurance claims?
- Do they have absenteeism or presenteeism issues?
- Do they have low employee satisfaction or participation in their wellness plan?
- Do employees suffer from preventable diseases?
- Are their workers' comp claims high? What are their DART and TRIR numbers and severity rates?
- Do new hires or a particular job group have higher injury rates?

Some of these answers can be deduced from digging into websites, as well as state employment and safety websites. Some may take networking or a phone call. Once you've gathered as much information as you can, use the formula in Chapter 6 to calculate the ROI your services will deliver.

When you approach a prospect armed with this information, you show them that you know what they need and that you are qualified and available to provide it. This makes you and your services irresistible.

This is real marketing—not brochures and heavy-handed sales pitches.

NETWORKING

When you're ready to connect with a company or prime contractor, it's better for everyone—and more comfortable for you— if you have the name of the right person to approach, the person who would be interested in what you have to say. It's even better if you've already met them.

To that end, as you set up your business, part of your marketing effort should be investing in becoming part of your industry and building a reputation for yourself and your company. You want to be involved; share information with colleagues; learn more about your clients and their businesses; and give potential clients the opportunity in a natural way to know you, what you do, and how you can solve their problems.

When you're just starting out, the easiest way to do this is to establish yourself through professional networks. For instance, if you're not already, become a member of the APTA. This gives you professional credibility and provides you with a host of opportunities to network with colleagues and vendors, who then can recommend you. It helps you stay current on developments in the profession. It allows you to meet people by attending the organization's state and national conferences. It also gives you access to all the people on the APTA's professional discussion boards, such as the Occupational Health and Safety Interest Group (OHsig) page, the private practice section (PPS), as well as ergonomic and safety networking pages.

For more extensive networking and positioning yourself and your business, the social media site LinkedIn lets you connect with both colleagues and potential clients without leaving your desk. If you're not a member now, join at the free membership level. Fill out your entire profile. Use the space to speak to potential clients and promote your services and benefits to them. Upload a picture and include full contact information and your web address.

Once on LinkedIn, connect to everyone you can. Search for those you've identified as your "ideal clients." Follow professional organizations, government agencies that deal with health care and insurance, and companies with on-site clinics. Connect with health and benefits directors, compensation and benefits directors, human resources directors, directors of operations, environmental health and safety managers, safety officers, and safety/trainer leaders. If you are looking to subcontract, connect to prime contractors.

Set five minutes aside a few mornings a week to look at your connections' posts and educate yourself about trends in their industry, as well as a company's particular needs. If you have something useful to say or an article to share, comment on their post and start a relationship. If a potential client shares several posts about employee retention, worker health, or injury prevention, take note that they might need your services. Luckily, because you're connected through LinkedIn, you have their contact information.

Use your posts to educate potential clients about on-site PT and to position yourself as an expert—someone who knows their stuff. I often post things like tips for keeping a workforce healthy or anecdotal stories that reinforce the benefits of on-site PT.

Boost these online efforts with in-person networking whenever possible. Investigate local health care organizations, as well as your state and local workers' compensation groups for insurance providers and physicians. Go to chamber of commerce, mentoring, or economic development events. By attending a mentoring session hosted by the Denver Business Journal, I connected with a healthcare reporter. The result was a great article in the DBJ focusing on my business model and its impact on patient care. Romano, Analisa "These Denver-area health care companies are sidestepping insurance" Denver Business Journal, March 22, 2023 https://ww.bizjournals.com/denver/news/2023/03/22/denver-health-care-companies-insurance.html

In your first year, try to attend at least one conference. Some that offer great programming—as well as the opportunity to meet potential clients—include the National Ergonomics Conference, the Safety Conference, the APTA Annual Conference, and the Self-Insurance Institute of America Conference.

Networking—taking every opportunity to get to know people who can use your services, as well as people who can recommend you and you can recommend—eliminates the fear factor in making the sale. It eliminates the learning curve for the potential client as well.

Most important, by meeting prospects first on neutral territory, you get a more honest impression of their needs. You get the chance to have an authentic, no-pressure discussion and get to know each other. Thus, should a "sale" seem appropriate, it will happen naturally from your learning what their challenges are and them learning about how you can help them. They are sold well before you make the ask.

SPEAKING OUT

For all the prospects out there that you don't have a chance to meet, the best way to reach them is to speak and write publicly. This also gives you added credibility in the minds of prospects you do know.

To be sure, the thought of public speaking or publishing can feel daunting. Again, I've found that if I frame it as helping others, getting them information they need, I don't feel so self-conscious. Keep in mind that it's about them—always them—not you.

If you don't have much experience speaking in public, start with smaller events. Local health care organizations, continuing education providers, local chambers of commerce, and other business organizations are always looking for speakers. Consider addressing their regular meeting or holding a workshop on an issue of importance to them. For instance, a chamber of commerce might be interested in general back injury prevention, where workers' compensation professionals would prefer a talk on how prevention programs increase productivity and save money. Whatever you talk about, you want them to see you as a trusted professional who has the answers they've been looking for.

If standing in front of an audience is too much at first, be a guest on a podcast. Make a list of podcasts your potential clients listen to. Note the content typically discussed. Then figure out topics in your area of expertise that would be of interest to their audience. Email the host or producer and pitch a topic to them. Start with less popular shows (those with fewer followers) and work your way up.

An even more low-key—but just as impactful—way to share your expertise with the world is writing a guest blog for a website or an article in a journal. Being published gives you instant credibility. So, again, figure out what your clients read and pitch your story ideas to that outlet. You'll be surprised how hungry they are for content.

One-stop shops—organizations that can get you in front of potential clients through myriad outlets (such as conferences, seminars, journals, online education, etc.)—include: The Self-Insurance Institute of America, Business Insurance, SafetyCenter.org, EHS Today, American Society of Safety Professionals, and NIOSH Total Worker Health Program. Organizations that can give you outlets and opportunities for professional credibility include the APTA, *Move* magazine, and your state safety association. Get on their websites and contact the person in charge of the outlet you want to participate in. **As of Spring 2023, both the APTA Private Practice Section and the Occupational Health Special Interest Group have created curriculums to facilitate direct to employer business and the growth of occupational health services. The Occupational Health Practitioner Certificate Program looks very promising so, check it out!**

WARM CALLING

Often we get so wound up in tending to "new prospects," we forget to take advantage of the people already in our corner. When I started my business, I personally contacted everyone I could think of—friends, vendors, colleagues—to tell them about McCallum Physical Therapy. In marketing, this technique is called "warm calling." The opposite of the cold call, you contact people you already know, fill them in on what you're up to (opening a new business!), and ask them to spread the word. Easy, right!

I found it really fun. It put me back in touch with people and allowed me to strengthen professional relationships I'd let slide. It was also successful. Immediately, I got leads, along with key introductions.

To start warm calling, make a list of one hundred people you know—professional contacts, friends, acquaintances. Break the list into sets of ten. Then over ten weeks, reach out to ten people a week in the way that's most appropriate for your relationship—email, phone call, and, for some, a handwritten note.

Personalize each communication. Ask them how they are. Remind them the last time you were in touch. For those you don't know well, remind them how you met. Then:

- Let them know you are starting a business—include your business name.
- Remind them of your credentials and experience.
- List the benefits of your services.
- Tell them who your ideal client is.
- Clearly, ask them to tell others and to refer you.

This is one of the easiest, most productive, and most pleasant techniques I use for generating leads and interest in my business.

As your business grows and you meet more people, add them to your warm list. Should you have a slow period or lose a big client, reaching back out to this list (though don't do it too often) can get you right back where you want to be. I reused my list to announce becoming certified as a Women-Owned Small Business (WOSB). I knew that designation would be important to current and potential clients who value supplier diversity.

THE COLD CALL

On occasion, you're going to discover a prospect who needs your help, and yet, you have no contacts at the company. When this happens, don't let the opportunity pass you or your prospective client by. Commit to a cold call.

If you can, find the name of the person in the company you need to talk to. Look on the company website or locate the annual report. If you can't find a name, pick up the phone, call the company's general line, and talk to the receptionist. I've found they're usually happy to direct me to the right person.

Once you make contact with the right person, keep your message short. Tell them who you are, give them a reason to talk to you—a benefit—and then invite them to talk now or later. Say something like: "Hi, John Carter. This is (your name) of (company name). My company provides injury prevention services for operations like yours. I have ideas that can save your company money. Do you have a moment to talk, or can we set up a short call in the near future?"

If they agree to talk, don't use that time to talk about yourself. Remember, sales is about service, solving a problem. I'm always ready with questions about their operation that lead them to realize their need for my services. I ask about current on-site care, new-hire injuries, extended time away for injured workers, and general employee health. I always end with a thank you and a request for permission to send them information. I tell them I will follow up in a few weeks—this keeps the connection ball in my court. If they blow me off, I send them information anyway and check back in a few months to see if they're more open to a discussion.

Several years ago, I worked with a marketing coach. My final training task was to do three cold-call visits in person. The first business had a receptionist who gave me the name and number of their occupational injury manager. The second business had a security desk I couldn't get past. So I told the security officer I was marketing my small injury prevention business and wasn't sure who to contact at the company. I asked if he had any suggestions. He looked up the safety manager and the assistant director of benefits. He didn't let me past the lobby, but I walked away with two solid contacts. Before entering the third business, I discovered I had a contact there—an HR manager. When I walked in, I asked the receptionist to message her, and she came out. She gave me her boss's email and said she'd let them know I'd be calling.

The lesson here is don't overthink cold calls. Most people want to help. And you know you're there to help their business. Though cold calls might feel uncomfortable, they're worth the effort.

MARKETING/EDUCATIONAL MATERIALS

As you network and connect, you need to have materials to reassure prospects that you're a professional and offer what they need. While business books and marketing gurus might have you believe you need a slick design, ads on the internet, or a content creator churning out pithy social media posts, all you really need is a few inexpensive pieces you can create yourself.

1. A capability statement

This very simple—but important—one-sheet lets potential clients know the scope of your services and how you help them meet their objectives. Use it to follow up after a meeting, as a handout at an event, or whenever anyone wants to know about your business.

As for design, consider using a template from your word processing software to give it some style. You want the reader to grasp the main points at a glance, so use bullet points freely. For now, your capability statement should include:

- Your company name and contact information
- Your credentials
- A photo of you
- A list of the services you offer (your capabilities!)
- The results that on-site PT delivers—health care savings, fewer workers' comp claims, higher productivity, etc.—with some statistics. (Later you can replace this with the results your company has achieved for clients.)

As you get clients, you can add their names or logos, a testimonial, or anything else you think would matter to potential clients.

Once you get the basics down, tailor this sheet to specifically speak to the needs and interests of whomever you are sending it to. I have three capability statements ready to go at all times. The first is a general statement (below) listing all my company's services, as well as information on how much those services reduce costs in the areas of injuries, presenteeism, and general rehab. My second one is targeted at health and benefits directors. My third is for safety managers. Feel free to use my general capability statement to help you create yours.

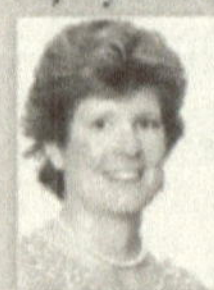

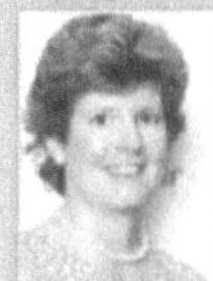

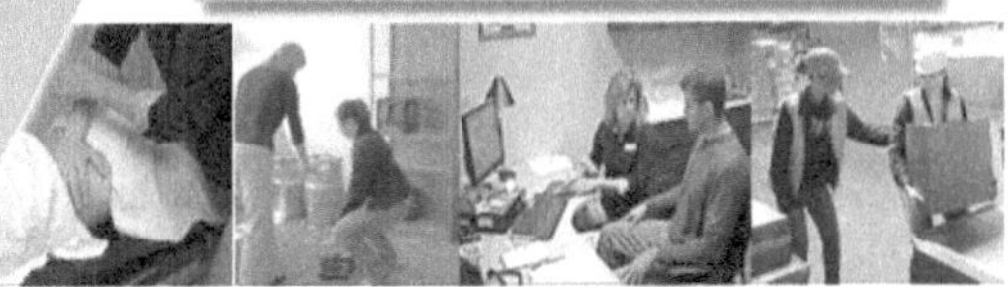

Established in 2015

State of Incorporation
Colorado

Office Location
Metro Denver

Minority Business
Woman Owned

WBENC certification

D & B: Upon Request

Primary NAICS codes:
621340, 621498, 621999

1. ON-SITE PT CAN TRIAGE DISCOMFORT/STRESSORS AND PREVENT THESE FROM BECOMING OSHA RECORDABLE

2. EMPLOYEES DO NOT HAVE TO LEAVE THE WORKSITE TO RECEIVE THE CARE THEY NEED

3. THE FURTHER ALONG ON THE HEALTH CONTINUUM A PROBLEM IS IDENTIFIED AND TREATED, THE MORE EXPENSIVE IT BECOMES

4. ON-SITE PT CAN HELP EASE WORRIES AND STRESSORS ABOUT INJURIES, AND IMPROVE YOUR EMPLOYEE EXPERIENCE

- Serving local corporate/manufacturing/distribution facilities in Colorado, for small, mid-size and large companies.

1. https://injuryfacts.nsc.org/work/work-overview/top-work-related-injury-causes/
2. https://www.osha.gov/dcsp/smallbusiness/safetypays/estimator.html
3. https://www.cpwr.com/sites/default/files/publications/DongEconomicConsequencesYouthSurveyKF.pdf
4. https://beebole.com/blog/cost-absenteeism-presenteeism/

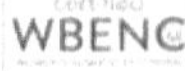
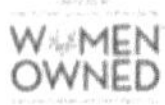
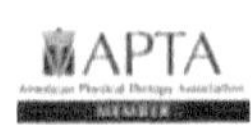
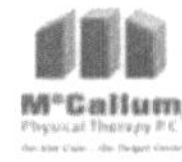

2. An elevator speech

When people ask you what you do, you want to be able to tell them succinctly and without hesitation. A good elevator speech—being able to describe your company in the time it takes an elevator to go a few floors (thirty seconds or so)—shows you are a professional who's clear on the service you deliver.

Your elevator speech should include your company name, who you serve, the problem you solve for them, and the results you get—touting your experience wherever possible. Your capability statement can help you with the language. My own elevator speech goes like this:

McCallum Physical Therapy provides companies with on-site physical therapy, including injury prevention, pre-employment screening, and treatment for employees, among other services. Companies provide this on-site benefit to their employees to keep them healthy. It's a cool way for employees to get the care they need and prevent injuries. As a therapist, I enjoy not working with insurance and having such impactful time with so many employees.

Once I give my speech, if the person I'm talking to could be a potential client, I ask them about their business—and then I listen. If it looks like I could help them, I ask to exchange business cards and if I can contact them to set up a time to talk further.

3. A business card

To be able to offer a business card, you must have one. It doesn't have to be fancy, but it does have to be professional—so don't print one off your computer. Online design and printing services are very affordable and offer professional-looking templates for cards. My first business card was from an online printing service and cost about $25 for 200.

Your business card should include your business's name, your name with your credentials, and your contact information with your website address. If you have a logo or a tagline, include it. But neither is necessary at this point.

4. A website

You must have a website. Having one adds to your legitimacy and credibility. It's the first thing a prospect looks for after meeting you.

Your site should be simple and straightforward. My site (mccallum-phyiscaltherapy.com) is three pages—welcome, services offered, and contact. Get ideas for content and design by checking out the websites of other on-site PT services. See what information they include. Note what you feel is missing that you might want on your site.

Web designers are plentiful. However, I built my first website myself to save costs. That was a decade ago. Today, it's even easier to put up a professional-looking site. Most online website builders walk you step-by-step through the entire process. Beware of "free" hosting, however. It means having their advertising all over your site, which isn't professional. I suggest paying the fee for an advertisement-free site. It's nominal. Mine runs about $100 a year for hosting and $10 to maintain my domain name.

5. A social media presence

Choose your social media carefully. It's too easy to waste time online. LinkedIn, as we've already discussed, is a good place to invest your efforts. But Facebook, Instagram, TikTok, or Twitter are not places your clients are likely to be, so you don't need to be there either.

That doesn't mean there won't come a time when one of them might make sense for your business. Technology moves fast. So monitor what's going on in social media, reconsider when necessary, and be prepared to tweak your strategy as called for.

As your business grows, you might consider hiring marketing professionals to upgrade the look of your marketing materials. After two years in business, I was ready to expand. About the same time, I attended an event and connected with people from a local business consulting group. They suggested my branding and marketing could be stronger and recommended a media consultant. Working with that consultant and the graphic artist he recommended, we came up with a custom logo, a tagline, and some promotional materials for my business that I still use today. I consider it money well invested. By the way, my tagline is: "On-Site Care . . . On-Target Costs."©

AFTER THE SALE

If you've laid the marketing groundwork as we outlined above, making the actual sale—asking your prospect if they want to work with you—will not be difficult. It will be a natural progression from the connecting and educating that's come before. At this point, you should know what your prospect's challenges are, and they should understand the benefits of hiring you. The only thing left should be writing up a contract (which we will go over thoroughly in Chapter 11) and signing it.

But just because the contract is signed doesn't mean your marketing effort is over. Once on the job, you want to deliver value and ensure the client knows it. So keep track of your work and outcomes, and again, use the formula from Chapter 6 to calculate what you've done for their company.

Once on the job, remember that your current client is your best prospect. Find places where your skills and knowledge can help even more. They already trust you. So they're open to your suggestions of how to improve their operation.

EVERYTHING IS MARKETING

Marketing your business is more an attitude than a specific set of actions. Everything is marketing. What you wear, the emails you send, what your invoices look like, how you answer the phone—all that sends a message to people about you and your business. So use it to your advantage. Because once they know you, it's these small things—not a big ad blast on Google— that convince potential clients to become clients and stay clients.

Marketing is knowing yourself, knowing your business, and, most of all, knowing the needs of the clients you serve best. It is indeed looking out for their interest 100 percent—and then some. As a PT, you're a natural at that.

···

EXERCISE:
Your Marketing Plan

···

Questions

1. In what areas of marketing do you already have good skills?

2. Which marketing activities look like the most fun to you? The most natural for you?

3. Which marketing activities seem the most difficult? (Consider hiring a professional to help with these.)

4. Are there wellness companies in your area that staff on-site PT clinics?

5. How will your business structure affect your marketing effort?

Activities

*   Map out your target area.

*   Define and then find your target market.

*   Create your prospect spreadsheet—with contact information, as well as whatever else you learn about your potential clients.

*   Create a to-do list and a calendar for completing your marketing materials.

*   Decide on which marketing activities are critical to promoting your business now. Make a to-do list and a calendar to get them done. Update regularly as you see which activities bring the most return for your business.

*   Review your professional networks and see where you might increase your presence. Then, do it.

11

PROPOSALS AND CONTRACTS

Before you start shopping for clients, however, you want to know how to put together your proposals and contracts. Obviously, each proposal and contract you prepare will be unique to your potential client (a company or prime contractor, depending on your business structure) and their needs. By taking the time now to thoroughly understand each document's purpose and craft some standard language and structure for each, you'll be able to produce them more efficiently, effectively, and accurately when the time comes.

Both proposals and contracts are about bringing clarity to a project for everyone. Proposals get people on the same page and address a potential client's areas of requested need. Contracts guarantee everyone understands what they've agreed to before work begins. The more precise your documents are, the better your client relationships will be, and the better your business will operate.

THE PROPOSAL

When you meet with a prospective client—whether as a prime yourself or looking to subcontract through them—you want the conversation to focus on them and their business (not you, not your business). You want to ask them what their needs are—not simply regarding on-site PT, but overall. You're working to uncover where and how you can best serve them—and there may be areas where on-site PT can help that they aren't aware of. To that end, you also want to understand their ultimate vision for their company. Only after you've listened to them attentively do you discuss where and how your services will solve their problems, advance their goals, and lower their costs. When done well, this initial meeting wraps up with your telling them you'll send a proposal outlining what you've discussed.

And that's all a proposal is—a repeat of this initial discussion in writing with more details, more clarity, and some numbers attached. You're not selling or pushing anything. You're giving them a written plan that spells out for both parties what you propose to do, why and how you're going to do it, the benefits they'll receive from your services, and your estimated fee.

For your prospect, the proposal is something they can hold in their hand, study, refer to, and share with other decision makers. For you, it's an opportunity to prove to them you understand what they need. It's a chance to show them—in bullet points wherever possible (you want to make it easy to scan)—that you have the ideas, the experience, the skill, and the professionalism to deliver it all. Your proposal puts down in black and white that you know how to address their issue, ease their workload, and in doing so, improve their company's performance all around.

For you, the actual writing of the proposal has the added benefit of making you thoroughly think through how you can best serve the client, where you might prevent problems for them, the amount of time and work this job is really going to demand from you, and what fair compensation would be. Again, there is nothing like having to put things in words to force us to get clear.

As you write the proposal, put yourself in your prospect's head. What's important to them? What do they need to know from you to make their decision to hire you or your practice? You want to toot your own horn but in a way that speaks to their success.

A typical proposal does this in six sections:

Section 1: Cover letter or email

This letter introduces the proposal. If you are sending the proposal via email (and that's how it's mostly done these days), this is the email you write and attach the proposal and any addendums to it in a PDF document. If you are sending this via snail mail (only do this if asked to), this letter is on its own page, separate from the proposal and addendums. Whichever you do, the letter should be no more than a few paragraphs.

Open the letter by reminding your prospect of your prior meeting and that you are following up with this proposal as promised. Say something positive about their business. Talk about the specific needs you discussed and how your on-site PT practice provides the solution. Then let them know the proposal is attached and the next step—which is that you will contact them. You want to take charge of making the next contact. You don't want to send off a great proposal only to be left wondering if they're going to act. (See sample cover letter below to get an idea of what you might write.)

Section 2: Scope of work

This section lays out the exact services your practice will deliver. You choose these services based on your discussion with the client, their stated goals, your research into their company, and your experience providing care—remember you're the expert here.

Make each item only as detailed as you think your prospect needs. If the proposal is being sent to a prime contractor, a safety manager, or third-party administrator, you won't need to define your services with as many specifics as you would for a company that's new to on-site wellness.

As with everything, think of your audience. You don't want to overwhelm or bore the prospect. But you do want to be sure they fully understand what you are proposing to deliver for them.

Section 3: Goals

In this third section, state in no uncertain terms the results they can expect from the scope of work you've outlined above. These benefits to your client should be specific, measurable, and directly speak to the goals the client brought up during your meeting. For instance, how much can they expect your services to reduce recordable injury rates, decrease primary care costs, and decrease rehabilitation costs? Use the formulas from Chapter 6 to help you think through and determine probable benefits and savings of your services.

Don't be shy here. They need to know the true value of having you on-site. While you shouldn't over-promise, you want to be sure they fully comprehend the return on investment you deliver.

Section 4: Timeline

This section lets the client know when everything happens. Write down the date you propose to begin providing services, how many days and hours you'll be on-site, and the length of the contract (how long it lasts—a year, three years, five years). Again, this is based on the discussion you had with the prospective client, as well as your expertise in knowing how many hours a week it will take for you to achieve what they want their on-site PT to achieve.

As for the duration of the contract, the longer it is, the better. A long contract gives you more time to make a difference for your client, as well as a more dependable cash flow for your business.

Section 5: Fees

This is usually where the prospective client's eyes go first. This section clarifies not only how much your services will cost but also how you bill. So you want to include:

- How you document your time
- The total cost per hour
- How often you invoice (usually monthly)
- When payment is due (typically within sixty days of receipt of invoice—remember you are a small business; you need to keep your revenue flowing)
- Any other terms you have.

Some on-site PT models choose to contract for a fee-for-service model that is structured like a rigid outpatient clinic fee schedule. Though simple and straightforward, this compensation model doesn't allow for the flexibility the company and the on-site PT need. You are dealing with human beings here. Injury and illness don't always resolve according to a fee schedule.

How I choose to be compensated is by negotiating for a set hourly fee and a guaranteed number of weekly hours. This model affords me a regular income I can count on (and my client can budget for) and the ability to schedule more time when more is needed. (You can see how I word this in the sample proposal below.) It just doesn't make financial sense to tie your payment to individual clinic sessions or to separate out each service you provide for a fee. This compensation model allows you to serve the client however best suits them, no matter what is needed.

A caveat: Some self-insured companies have a high-deductible health plan and provide their employees with a health savings account (HSA) with matching funds. This is helpful when an employee has high health care expenses. However, there are tax implications to this. So, in such a situation, you, as the on-site PT, may be required to set a fee for treatment, whether or not that's how your compensation is structured in your contract. All you need to understand about this right now is that a high deductible/HSA plan will not affect the fee you negotiate with your client. How and what you are paid is between you and the self-insured company. But if you do end up working with a client who has a high-deductible plan, you should check with your business attorney and the company's insurance representative to determine your insurance billing responsibilities as an independent contractor.

Section 6: Client obligation

Up to this point, your proposal has been about describing what you're responsible for as the on-site PT. This section is about what your client's obligations will be—what they need to do so you can do what you do. For instance, you might ask that they provide space for you; specific equipment (which we'll go over thoroughly in Chapter 12, and which you'll detail in an addendum to the proposal); regular communication to their workforce about you and clinic services; and regular meetings to discuss clinic progress and strategize when needed.

SAMPLE COVER LETTER AND PROPOSAL

I've included a cover letter and proposal samples, so you can see what these documents look like. Both were created for a client with a solid knowledge of on-site wellness and PT, so not a lot of description was needed. As you create your proposals, however, remember to speak to your particular client. What do they know? What do they need to know?

> SAMPLE COVER LETTER:

Dear Ms. Smith,

I enjoyed meeting with you on Tuesday and learning more about ACME Industries. It was evident how important it is to you that your employees are well cared for. Your concern about the rising cost of insuring them and keeping them healthy is well placed—making your decision to invest in on-site physical therapy a sound one. As we discussed, study after study has shown on-site PT to decrease injuries and OSHA-recordable incidents, as well as overall health care costs.

Attached is the proposal you requested for McCallum Physical Therapy to provide services at your location. I will be in touch in a few days to see if you have any questions. I'm excited for this opportunity to enhance ACME's overall workforce wellness and profitability.

Kind regards,

Chris McCallum PT, DPT

McCallum Physical Therapy

(Add your contact information below your name—email and phone number—for easy reference.)

SAMPLE PROPOSAL:

PROPOSAL

(Date)

TO: Jane Smith, ACME Industries

FROM: Dr. Chris McCallum, PT, DPT

FOR: On-Site Physical Therapy Program

Scope of Work

McCallum Physical Therapy, P.C. will provide the following on-site:

- Injury prevention services
- One-on-one job coaching (*You may wish to add details here.*)
- Post-offer pre-employment testing program—including annual job analysis and validation of job functions and test
- OSHA-allowable first aid services
- Office ergonomics (*If your client is unfamiliar, you'll need a description here.*)

Goals To Be Attained

- Decrease OSHA-recordable injuries by 10 percent as compared to (*the previous year*)
- Decrease costs associated with primary care and rehab for workers' compensation injuries as compared to (*the previous year*)

Timeline

- Begin service on (*date*)
- Therapist will be on-site 3 days per week for 6 hours each day between the hours of 7:00 a.m. and 7:00 p.m. Exact hours to be

determined based upon safety needs, operation needs, and client preference.

- This will be an annual contract.

Pricing

- Services will be documented at 15-minute increments up to 18 hours per week.
- The cost is $XXX per hour.
- Hours will be documented and invoiced monthly to the client
- Payment is due 60 days after invoice date.
- If more time is requested by client, this hourly rate will be renegotiated if needed.

Client Obligation

- Provide PT with 10x10 foot space with privacy for clinic area.
- Purchase necessary equipment for clinic, such as treatment table, small desk, theraband, and job-testing equipment. See addendum A for recommended purchase list, with a total price of no more than $5,000.
- Facilitate postings and advertisements of PT clinic services on the property.
- Meet monthly for clinic update and strategy sessions.

In addition to the equipment addendum, I also attach my capabilities statement and a brochure, so they can read more about my practice.

Whatever word processing program you're using, create some personalized stationery from one of its templates. Be sure your company name and all your contact information are on it (and your logo, if you have one). Use this "stationery" for the first page of your proposal and any addendums. Before sending anything out, be sure to proof carefully. You don't want to seem careless. You want your proposal to reflect the professional you are.

NEGOTIATIONS

Proposals are a starting point. From here, expect to negotiate. The more you and your prospect can hammer out and agree to before writing the contract, the smoother the actual closing of the deal will go, as well as the job itself.

Unlike a brick-and-mortar clinic, every aspect of how you work is up for negotiation—your range of services, your hours, your compensation. And "negotiation" doesn't mean you give in to what your client wants. It means you both have goals for your businesses, you both have a say, and you work together to come to an agreement that suits everyone.

For instance, you've probably heard somewhere along the way that the cost of having an employee is 30 to 50 percent more than their hourly salary. Keep this in mind as you negotiate your fee. If you want to net $50 an hour, your cost per hour needs to be 30 to 50 percent higher than that value to cover Medicare, Social Security, income taxes, liability and commercial business insurance, unemployment insurance, workers' compensation insurance, and other expenses. Talk with your accountant about what your revenue needs to be to achieve your take-home goals.

Usually, after reviewing the proposal, the prospect has some questions, a few ideas of their own, and maybe some things they forgot to bring up in your first meeting. Once again, your job is to listen hard. If their request makes sense, incorporate it. If you think they are making a mistake—for instance, they don't want a service you strongly believe they need—speak up.

Remember, they're looking to you to guide them. If they still decide against what you recommend, you get to decide if you can move forward without it and still provide the level of service you want. If you can, note the service in question—and be prepared to propose your recommendation again once they trust you more and the need for the service they declined becomes more evident to them. You can always build change into the contract by saying, "If a change in services is requested or required, both parties will agree to said change and on any increase in fees required." Then, should you need to make a change, you simply create an addendum to the contract reflecting these changes.

Building change into the negotiation gives the potential client a sense of control over future services. They don't feel like they have to buy it "all" up front. It gives them a chance to ease into the new services, see the results, and become invested in you and the results your company provides.

The point here is everything is open for discussion. Listen to your client. But also respect what you bring to the table. You deserve to work in a way that results in the best outcomes for your clients, as well as proper compensation for you.

THE CONTRACT

With negotiations finished and terms agreed on, it's time to put your agreement into a binding legal document—also known as a contract.

You've been exposed to and signed many contracts in your life. Any time you've "agreed to terms" on a website, at the doctor's office, opening a bank account, you've entered into a contract. Most of us don't read the long, boring, tiny print that we initial and sign our names to. The legal nature of the writing makes it difficult to understand. However, as a business owner, it's important you not only read but understand that tiny print.

Whenever you provide services or secure services as a professional, you should have a contract. A good contract not only protects you from those with bad intentions, but it also prevents misunderstandings in the first place. With a good contract, whenever there's a disagreement, both parties have only to turn to that piece of paper to see what was agreed to, what wasn't, and straighten things out from there. A good contract removes awkwardness from the relationship. It ensures details are taken care of and responsibilities are assigned before you start work. Contracts also come in handy when personnel changes occur. Instead of having to explain what I do over and over again to a new services manager, account manager, or client liaison, I simply refer them to my contract.

To accomplish these good things for you and all parties, however, contracts must be precise and thorough. There are a lot of "what if" scenarios to think about when you enter into an agreement. That's why it's best to craft your contracts with the help of an attorney—they're experts at thinking about what could go wrong.

When I met with my attorney about my first client contract, I handed her what I'd written. Overall, it was pretty good. But quickly, she honed in on a sentence that read: "50 hours/week for all professional PT services."

To me that sounded fine and correct. But my attorney pointed out that the contract had no provision for normal fluctuations in demand. What happened if there was less traffic or work for me to do than fifty hours a week? What exactly constituted "professional PT services" anyway? Would I get paid less if I did not provide fifty hours' worth of work? And what time of day would I be expected to provide those fifty hours? All around the clock? Whenever my client called?

In the end, she changed my contract to read: "Up to 50 hours per week of professional services, provided during typical clinic daytime hours." In the scope of work section, we spelled out specifically what those services would entail. The new language made clear that there was no penalty to me if some weeks there were fewer than 50 hours needed. The phrase "typical clinic daytime hours" also limited my on-site shifts to the hours of 6:00 a.m. at the earliest to 6:00 p.m. at the latest. This did not prevent me from doing work outside of those hours when needed, such as performing a job analysis with an employee that worked the night shift. This language did set the expectation of when we would be typically open and allowed me to change the schedule as needed to meet the client's needs.

My attorney reminded me that since I'm not an employee, the client cannot tell me what time to arrive or leave. As an independent contractor, I can change the schedule as needed to maximize clinic utilization and make it as easy as possible for employees to access the service. In that same vein, while the contract language prevents me from having to work after 6:00 p.m., it doesn't prevent me from doing so if I choose. If I need to do a job observation or ergonomics in the production area in the evening, I can decide to. Those things are needed sometimes. Thanks to my attorney, my contract allows me to serve my client the way I know is best.

When I'm ready to write a contract, I start with an old contract. I change whatever particulars need changing to address my new situation. Then I get my attorney to review it before handing it to the second party for signing.

PARTS OF A CONTRACT

In general, the sections of your contract are much the same as the sections in your proposal without the goals (unless you can completely guarantee outcomes, they don't belong in a legally binding document.) Also, each section has a few more technical and specific details added.

For instance, the contract will likely include information on the type of professional who will deliver the services (PT, PTA, ATC, etc.). Under "Terms" might be clauses about state licensing for professional purposes, as well as tax purposes. There may be a noncompete clause, as well as information addressing insurance requirements. (Large companies usually expect $1 million to $3 million in liability and commercial business insurance.)

Because it's a legal agreement, the language will be more formal than the proposal. However, the document itself won't necessarily be long. For my smaller clients, contracts run about a page. For larger clients—where I do more and place employees—contracts can run from two to four pages.

Just to give you an idea of how an on-site PT contract reads, below is my standard prime-contractor-to-client contract:

SAMPLE CONTRACT

Scope of Work and Payment Agreement between McCallum Physical Therapy, P.C. (Company) and NAME (Client)

1. *Company will provide professional physical therapy services on-site at Client location (ADDRESS).*
2. *Company will provide all services with a Colorado State Licensed Physical Therapist in good standing. The Company will provide a portable massage table, massage and cleaning products, and exercise equipment as needed for Client.*
3. *Services will be agreed upon by both parties before initiation.*
4. *Fee: $X/hour for first two hours on-site each visit. If more than two hours are spent on-site, the fee is $X-15%/hour for remainder of that day. (This two-tiered billing structure covers my transportation*

costs but doesn't overcharge the client since I drop it down after two hours on-site).

> *a. Paid services include massage, physical therapy evaluation and treatment, ergonomics, lifting/body mechanics training, and exercise/self-care instruction.*
>
> *b. Complimentary services that may be needed include job observation and documentation off the clock with personalized exercise programs.*

5. *Current treatment days will be either Tuesday or Thursday. Each treatment will last between 30 and 60 minutes, as care needs indicate.*

6. *All medical records and forms will be the property of McCallum Physical Therapy, P.C. and will be confidential. All medical records will be protected under HIPAA, HITECH provisions, and will be secured accordingly. Client has the right to knowledge of which employees utilized the service, but no other information about the session or client condition.*

Client agrees to pay for services documented (at fee stated in #4 above) and invoiced to client.

Weekly hours will be reported and will be invoiced biweekly.

Signature, The Company, Date   *Signature, The Client, Date*

The Employee Contract

My subcontractor-to-prime contractor contract is similar to my prime-to-client contract—tweaked to suit the job, of course. When I hire employees, however, that contract is very different.

If you choose to hire employees in the future, you want a contract with them to be airtight. Most states have many laws surrounding the employer-employee relationship. You need to know what they are, understand them, and ensure they're incorporated into your employer/employee contract where appropriate. In other words, keep your lawyer close as you create this contract.

Items you want to be sure are addressed and considered include:

The Job

- Clearly stating that the other party is an employee and what that means legally for them and for you, the employer.
- What services they will be expected to provide and when. For instance, if the employee is responsible for handling payments or collecting and documenting payments, make sure this is clearly spelled out in the contract.
- What licensing they must hold and that it's their responsibility to keep it current.
- The time frame of when they will be expected to work—if that is pertinent to how you run your business. (I do not state a time frame in my employee contract, because I want flexibility. Also, my contract with my clients stipulates regular business hours. So, scheduling hasn't been an issue with my employees.)
- The site to which they will be assigned—again, only if that is pertinent to the way you run your business.

The Benefits

- The rate of their pay and how they are paid—including straight or overtime options, shift differentials, holiday pay, or other pay structures. (All my employees are part time and so are paid a straight hourly wage.) My attorney recommended getting all the employees signed up for direct deposit for their payroll. This eliminates the need for me to write and send out checks, which takes the pressure off me to meet a delivery deadline.

- A description of the benefits they receive, such as tax-deferred IRA contribution, vacation days, sick days, etc. Know your state's requirements for any sick days you must provide, Family and Medical Leave Act (FMLA) insurance you or the employee must fund, and the like.

Expectations

- Tardiness and absenteeism policy. What constitutes each? What are the established rules around each? What happens if rules are abused or broken?
- Drug policy
- Professional behaviors. Spell out what that means—i.e., professional appearance, professional demeanor, no disparaging comments, etc.
- Confidentiality agreement
- Noncompete clause for a period of six months to a year—with an associated fine if this is broken.

Termination

- Provide instructions for how both parties can terminate the contract. For instance, I request the professional courtesy of four weeks' notice. This allows me time to find a replacement. In turn, I agree to provide a four-week notification in advance of termination or ending of the contract.

The above is in no way an exhaustive list of what goes into an employer/employee contract. But it gives you an idea of the scope of matters that should be addressed. You can plainly see why you want someone with legal expertise to help you craft such a document. A lot can go wrong with employing people without a good contract, so much goes right when you have a good one.

While this doesn't go in the contract, it's important to note that your state labor board, workers' compensation insurance, and professional liability insurance will require that you inform them of your total number of employees and full-time equivalents. This will dictate your unemployment, workers' compensation, and liability insurance fees. When you gain or lose an employee, you need to change the policies to stay accurate.

Below are the primary points in the employment contract I typically use when I on-board an employee. Colorado is an at-will employment state, with exceptions. As I said, your state will have its own laws, which must be considered and reflected in the content of your contract.

SAMPLE EMPLOYEE CONTRACT

EMPLOYMENT AGREEMENT

This agreement for employment is made between the (Employer) McCallum Physical Therapy, P.C. and the (Employee) Candidate's name.

Contract legal terminology: Employer wishes to hire employee and vice versa, based upon the terms of this agreement.

TERMS

Clear Description of the Job Duties, including weights required to lift, necessary tasks, and regulations that need to follow.

A. <u>Name of Position</u>. Employee shall be employed in the capacity of: Physical Therapist.

B. <u>Essential Job Functions and Duties</u>. The essential job functions or duties of this position are as follows: Manual physical therapy, use of modalities, use of patient-specific therapeutic exercise, able to safely lift up to 50 lbs. (rarely) and 20 lbs. (frequently), document using APTA-approved format, manage patient care and recovery, assist with return-to-work planning, provide ergonomic assessments, schedule patients, and ensure proper billing/charging.

C. <u>Additional Responsibilities</u>. Other duties that are part of normal business duties, such as scheduling, communication, and cleaning, as well as such other reasonable duties as may be assigned from time to time by Employer.

D. <u>Place and Hours of Employment</u>. Employee agrees that his/her duties shall be rendered at the agreed upon location(s) set by the Employer. Part-time work is expected from the Employee.

I. SALARY/HOURLY PAY RATE

A. <u>Base Compensation</u>. Employee shall receive a base pay of DOLLARS ($X) per hour. Employer shall deduct or withhold from compensation all sums required for federal income, social security taxes, and all state and/or local taxes.

B. <u>Expense Reimbursement</u>. The Employee shall not be entitled to reimbursement of any reasonable expenses related to work unless prior approval is received in writing from the Employer.

II. BENEFITS

A. <u>Vacation</u>. Employer's vacation policy is as follows: Vacation for part-time employees will be unpaid. Thirty-day notice required for approval. Up to 50 hours off per year for vacation reasons.

III. TERMINATION

This is an "At-Will" employment agreement "At-Will" is defined as either Employee or Employer being able to discontinue the agreement with or without cause or notice.

IV. COMMITMENT

A. <u>Nondisclosure of Proprietary or Confidential Information</u>. Employee agrees to not disclose information that is confidential or proprietary relating to McCallum Physical Therapy, P.C., our patients, or the Client we serve. Unauthorized disclosure is considered a breach of this Employment Agreement.

B. <u>Non-Solicitation of Employer's Customers</u>. Employee agrees that for a period of six months following termination of Employee's employment, for any reason whatsoever, Employee will not solicit customers or clients of Employer.

C. <u>Non-Recruit Covenant</u>. Employee agrees not to recruit any of Employer's employees for the purpose of any outside business either during or for a period of six months after Employee's term of employment with Employer terminates.

V. ARBITRATION

Disputes to be resolved using current arbitration rules applicable to Colorado employment laws and resolutions will be considered binding.

VI. LIMITATION OF DAMAGES

This section relates to employees breaching the employment-related obligations, neglect, or laws that negatively affect the Employer. It will state a financial value or salary equivalency that the employee would be responsible for.

VII. ATTORNEYS' FEES AND COSTS

Prevailing party entitled to recovery of reasonable attorney fees related to the litigation.

VIII. MISCELLANEOUS PROVISIONS

A. <u>Notices</u>. Notices relating to this Agreement shall be sent to the following addresses:

For Employer: McCallum Physical Therapy, P.C.
                      ADDRESS
For Employee: NAME
                      ADDRESS

B. <u>Entire Agreement</u>. This is the whole agreement, which includes addendums A and B (etc.) as attached. There are no other agreements in place for this Employer-Employee relationship.

C. <u>Severability</u>. If something in this agreement is determined to be unenforceable, all other items in this contract are still in effect.

D. <u>Choice of Law, Jurisdiction, and Venue</u>. This agreement will be defined per all laws of the State of CO, and the parties agree to the venue of County Name, State of CO for all actions on this agreement.

IN WITNESS WHEREOF, Employer and Employee have both executed this Agreement as of April 01, 2015.

EMPLOYER   EMPLOYEE

___________________   ___________________

Christine McCallum   Name

President, McCallum Physical Therapy, P.C.

Of course, you won't be rigid about everything in the contract. If an employee needs a few days off and tells you a week ahead instead of the four weeks stipulated in the contract and it works with the scheduling, of course you are going to make it happen. But the contract is there in case it doesn't work for you. The contract keeps the control with you.

EASY NOW OR HARD LATER

Somewhere in life, I came across the phrase "hard now, easy later," which to me is what proposals and contracts are about in a nutshell. Those who are lazy about their proposals and contracts end up in business relationships with a lot of misunderstandings that result in added stress, anger, passive-aggressive behaviors, or worse, not getting paid your worth. But when you invest the time to get your proposals and contracts as right as you can from the start, everything that flows from that effort is better and more rewarding for everyone all around.

If only all our relationships came with a contract. I'm kidding, of course. But there's an ease that comes with knowing what's expected, what to expect, and what the rules are before heading into any relationship. In addition, that period between proposal and contract, where you negotiate disagreements and figure out how to handle potential rough patches together, works to build understanding and trust between you and your new client.

In his poem, *Mending Wall*, Robert Frost famously wrote: "Good fences make good neighbors." In that same vein, good proposals and contracts make good client relationships. They are the foundation of a great business. Take them seriously and they will serve you, your clients, and your business well.

EXERCISE
Prepare Your Templates

Questions

1. Which contracts do you see yourself needing?
2. Do you have questions about contracts to ask your lawyer? Your CPA?

Activities

- Figure out what you need to know from a potential client and create a client-interview template.
- Write out a template for your proposal cover letter and your proposal.
- Write out a template for any of the contracts you think you'll need.
- Have your attorney review your template.

12

—

RUNNING YOUR SHOP

You're in the home stretch. You know what you need to do to open your on-site PT practice and secure clients. All that's left is putting the equipment and systems in place to run your operation.

As the owner of an on-site PT practice, you work in two spaces: your home office and your client's on-site clinic. You, of course, are responsible for your home office and everything in it. Your client is responsible for the cost of the space, furniture, equipment, and supplies needed to run your on-site station. It's up to you, however, to inform your client about what you need, order the supplies, and operate your on-site station.

AT HOME

When it comes to setting up your home office, here's a word of caution learned the hard way from my own experience: When I started out, I decided to cut corners here to save money. I decided my "office" would be my kitchen table. My kitchen chair could work as an office chair. I could use the same computer for my business as I used for my personal life. You get the picture. While it seemed like a frugal move at the time, it ended up costing me in ways I did not anticipate.

For instance, it cost me in time. Whenever anyone came to the house, I had to clean off the kitchen table (i.e., move my entire office) and then put it back together when I needed to work again—no easy task. This arrangement also took its toll in the form of increased anxiety. With all this shifting/shuffling, nothing had a permanent place. I'm a neat and orderly person for the most part, yet my business was always in a jumble. I was constantly looking for things. On top of all that, I developed back pain thanks to my poor ergonomic setup. I preach regularly to my clients that kitchen chairs are fine for eating cereal or sipping coffee and reading the paper, but they are not good for sitting for hours at a stretch working on spreadsheets and documents. Of course I knew this, but my focus was elsewhere, and I didn't practice what I preached.

However, the highest and most surprising cost of not investing in a proper space and equipment was that it made me feel like less of a business owner. By treating my business like a side hustle—like something I squeezed into my life—I wasn't giving it or my efforts the respect they deserved. This affected my attitude for sure, and I worried that all the chaos affected my performance. All this is to encourage you to be smarter than I was. Give yourself permission to create a proper home office.

If you must combine some parts of your home life with your office life to keep expenses down at first, go ahead. Don't let that stop you from opening your business. But understand the drawbacks of that setup. Know that the sooner your business has the space and equipment to operate well, the better for your business, your stress level, and you. As an added incentive to do this soon rather than later, remember that everything you purchase for your business can be a tax deduction—the clearer those lines are drawn, the bigger the savings and the fewer the problems you will have justifying the deduction.

Here are the barebones minimum things you need to get your home office up and running well:

1. Space and furniture

If you're able, designate a whole room in your home for your business—preferably a room with a door. If that's impossible right now, at least find a space that's out of the way of normal household activity—a place where you can be alone, concentrate, and keep the things you need around you. You want a place where you don't have to move your files, your papers, or your computer when people come over. You want a place that allows for a business-time mindset.

For furnishings, start with a desk (student size is fine). You need at least a two-drawer filing cabinet—you want to keep your business files separate from your personal files. A bookcase is handy. And don't skimp on investing in a quality office chair—as a PT you know it is worth it.

2. Hardware

Because you work in two spaces, you want devices that can travel with you when needed. Some PTs like using a tablet when they're on-site. But I find tablets cumbersome to type on, so I use a laptop. Whatever type of computer you choose, be sure that it has enough memory to run ergonomic spreadsheets. If possible, it should also have a touch screen. Touch screens make filling out forms so much easier—and as you know, PTs fill out a lot of forms. If the computer is capable of taking photos, that's a plus. If not, your phone can work just as well. And of course, your computer should be able to be locked when you're not using it.

This may surprise you, but you need a printer in your home office. Because of HIPAA laws and the HITECH Act, anything you send electronically must be encrypted—especially EMRs and personal health information (PHI). Some clients' computers may not be set up to read encrypted file transfers. In such cases, you want to have the capability to print/scan records to meet the security requirements for transfer.

If you have to buy a printer, consider buying one that has a fax machine function. Just as EMRs have almost made printers obsolete, they have also made faxing not as common as it once was in the medical world. Still, sometimes there is a need. So as long as you're purchasing a printer, it might as well have that capability.

3. Software

As for the software to run your business, you need an office suite—such as Microsoft Office or Home—that allows you to create documents, read PDFs, and create and edit spreadsheets. Also, as we've discussed in previous chapters, you must have a good accounting software. The software should be able to connect securely to your business bank account and generate professional-looking invoices that can be customized with your logo. This allows for automatic tracking of expenses, income, and customer payments—saving you loads of time and making it easy to compile your tax data or send to your accountant.

There are PT-specific accounting programs out there. However, the accounting for running an on-site PT business is much simpler than operating a brick-and-mortar clinic. I've always just used QuickBooks and found it does everything I need. Before you invest in accounting software, ask friends who are small-business owners what they use and recommend or ask your tax professional.

Most software packages these days give you a choice between a monthly subscription or purchasing the software outright. Though easier on the cash flow, software subscriptions usually only allow you to back up your work to their cloud. I opt for buying and owning the software. I feel safer backing up all my documents for my business—especially my banking ledger—on a device I control, so this works better for me.

4. A business bank account

Do not mix your personal funds with your business funds. Let me repeat that: Do not mix your personal funds with your business funds. You must have a separate bank account for your business. To get started, all you need is a small business checking account with a business credit card linked to that account. Be sure your business account also has a direct-deposit option, as most companies use electronic checks to pay their invoices these days.

As my business has grown, I've incorporated a credit card payment system into my banking because some clients prefer to pay this way. If you choose to allow credit card payments, be aware that it typically costs you around 3 percent of whatever is charged on it, and there is a standard monthly fee. Be sure to account for this cost-of-doing-business when deciding the fees you will charge your client.

5. Connection

To make this all work, of course, you need internet and phone service in your home office. Your internet connection needs to be fast and reliable—otherwise both you and your clients will become frustrated quickly. If that's not possible at your house—and it's still not in many rural areas—you might look into coworking spaces nearby that have fast internet.

You also need good cell phone service. Even if you have a landline, most of your clients are going to connect with you by cell. After all, that's the phone that's always with you. And these days, most clients and patients prefer to communicate via text. If you do use the same cell phone for work as you do for your personal calls (it's best not to, but most small-business owners I know—including me—do), be sure your recorded message is professional, not personal.

These are the very basics for your home office. They should be all you need to get up and running.

ON-SITE

Though every on-site clinic is unique, the basics of the on-site setup are pretty much the same. As the person in charge of your client's on-site station, it's up to you to figure out what supplies and systems you need to guarantee a smooth operation. Here are some items to consider as you think through your on-site setup:

1. The on-site location

The client provides both office space and treatment space for the on-site clinic at their location and at no cost to you. (Don't let them try to rent you space. But also know that in many clinics, the office and treatment space may be the same space.) Your contract with them should specify where your clinic will be located and how large it will be. You want a space that's easily accessible for employees and big enough that you can perform your work. In my career, I have worked in every size space, from an 8 ft. x 8 ft. cubicle to a full PT clinic (15 ft. x 40 ft.) with my own office, attached to a fitness center. By the way, I do not recommend that 8 ft. x 8 ft. cubicle. You need at least 10 ft. x 10 ft.

2. On-site documentation and secure internet

Since you must document treatments and complete consent forms via EMR while on-site, you need a small desk and chair for your space. If the client makes a computer available to you, that's best. If not, you can use your own laptop or tablet.

Whatever computer you use, it should have enough processing speed and memory to access an online EMR system. You will need to purchase a small-business EMR plan for one or two therapists. This small plan—which doesn't cost much—is essential. If you have more than one client, you can separate them into different "clinics" easily. That's all you need. Since you don't bill insurance, you don't need all the Medicare/insurance bells and whistles or the compliance extras that come with the bigger plans. (Just a reminder: If you download anything to your computer to upload into the EMR, remember to delete the file from the computer to keep the information secure.)

These days, you can do almost all the documentation and office work online. However, when you are on-site, you may still need access to a scanner, printer, and copier for forms or to print out instructions for patients.

3. Equipment

Part of your proposal and your contract to prospective clients is a supply list (with costs) to stock their on-site clinic. They pay for whatever you need to operate on their site. However, you do the actual ordering and re-ordering.

I keep a master list of basic supplies—along with current costs. This way, when I need to create a proposal or contract or need to reorder anything, my research has been done. With proposals and contracts, I find this master list is also a helpful checklist that keeps me from forgetting things.

The equipment you need for a particular site is determined by the service you're providing to the client. Obviously, as your services increase, your supply list will grow as well. Using the following (comprehensive) checklist can help you determine what you need to put on your supply master list and in your subsequent proposals and contracts:

For Manual Treatment:
- Massage table (1)
- Face cradle papers (100)
- Pneumatic stool (1)
- Massage cream (1)
- Pulse massager (1)
- Pillow (2)
- Paper pillowcases (100)
- Disposable shorts (50)
- Disposable towels (100)
- Reflex hammer (1)
- Goniometer (2)
- Gloves (1 box of 100)
- Hand sanitizer (1)
- Table sanitizer spray or wipes (1)

For Exercise:
- Foam roller (1)
- Theraband, small (1 roll, 3 colors)
- Putty (4)
- Taped tennis balls (1)
- Theracane (1)

- Stretching/yoga strap (2)
- Timer (1)

For Modalities:
- Hydrocollator, small (1)
- Hot pack pads to match (4)
- Small freezer (1) with soft-sided ice packs (4)
- Instant ice and hot packs (25 each)
- Kinesio tape (bulk, precut)
- Athletic tape (12 rolls)
- Portable NMES/IFC (1)
- Electrodes (20 sets of 4)
- Scissors (2)
- BioFreeze, mini packs (100)

For First Aid:
- Gauze bandages (1 pack)
- Elastic bandage wrap (1 three inch, 4 six inch)
- Adhesive bandage for fingers, etc. (1 box)
- Antibiotic ointment (1 box of individual packets)
- Self-adherent wrap (2 two inch, 2 one inch)
- Non-rigid wrist and ankle wraps (2 each)

For pre-employment testing and work conditioning:
- Lifting crate, capacity up to 100 lbs. (1)
- Adjustable shelves, 8 ft. height (1 set)
- Cuff weight set, 100 lbs. (1)
- Hand weights, varied weights up to 25 lbs. (1 set)

- Push-pull force dynamometer (1)
- Grip dynamometer (1)
- Pinch gauge (1)
- Tape measure, 25 ft. (1)
- Side-carry toolbox (1)
- Work gloves (1 pair)
- Heart rate monitor (1)
- Blood pressure monitor (1)

Don't expect your client to be familiar with many of these items. To help my clients make more sense of the supplies I need, I present them in "packages" that correlate with the services offered. For instance, I have a regular OSHA first aid supply list, as well as prevention training, work conditioning, pre-employment testing, and regular PT treatment lists.

As you begin to get your on-site station ready for patients, set up an account with your preferred vendor that requires your client's approval. That way you can order what you need and have your client billed directly.

4. Systems for Care

I had a business coach once who said that a stressor indicates a need for a system improvement. You want to prevent as much stress as you can by putting in place good systems for your on-site clinic and patient care before you're open for business. As you envision your workflow and favored habits—how you want things to go and what you'll need to make that happen—the systems you need to put in place will become clearer.

That said, here are a few areas where a good system can make everyone's experience better:

a) Appointment scheduling system: With on-site care, the majority of your patients will schedule their appointments and see you on the same day. Phone apps can make this process easy for both of you. You might also consider using a QR code—the employee simply scans the code and signs up for an available appointment. If neither of these systems is practical for your patient base, a good old-fashioned handwritten sign-up sheet can work just fine. Whatever system you choose to use, if part of your on-site services includes employee observation, be sure to block some time on the schedule to be in the work areas observing employees at work.

b) Patient intake system and required forms: You want to have a system for onboarding patients. A good system ensures all necessary steps and paperwork gets done. To create such a system, ask yourself a series of questions: What happens after a patient schedules an appointment? What do you need to do pre-appointment? What do they need to do? What forms do you need/want to have—HIPAA privacy notice, consent-for-care form, PT intake and medical history form, etc. Do they fill out forms online before they arrive or at the on-site clinic? Don't be afraid of getting this wrong. Simply make some decision about how you want to onboard patients, see how your system works, and tweak as needed.

c) Outside resources system: An on-site clinic does not have the equipment or expertise to treat every issue your patients will present with. You want to be prepared for those situations and have a list of trusted referrals ready. Referral relationships take work to establish but can work in your favor as well as the patient's. You appear knowledgeable and professional when you refer out correctly, and you may get more business from these external sources. On that list be sure to have the occupational medical clinic where employees should go for work-related injuries that require medical care. This information will come from the client, and the procedures for using that clinic will be clearly laid out by the client. Other external referrals may include a nearby PT who can do dry needling or other treatments you aren't able to perform on-site, as well as a gym, a mental health provider (this might be part of the employee's health benefits plan), and any other providers your patients might need.

d) An exercise prescription system: You can prescribe exercises the old-fashioned way—with printed instructions, stick drawings for illustrating form, and written notes crammed in the margins. Or you might consider systematizing your exercise prescriptions by using an online exercise program platform. These platforms make it easy for you to create custom home exercise programs (HEPs) for your patients. Most offer clear instructions, along with demonstration videos patients can watch at home as they go through their HEPs, and trackers, so both you and your patient can monitor progress. For me, these online exercise program platforms have elevated my HEP prescriptions and improved patient outcomes.

e) An hour tracking system: Even though your contract lays out how many hours you're expected to have the on-site clinic open each week, you want to keep an accurate record of those hours along with what you accomplished in them. Having a system here prevents you from putting this on the back burner until you can't remember when you were where and what you did. The more conscious you can become about what you do and how you do it, the better you will be at it. It's also invaluable data to have when it's time to renegotiate your contract with your client or plan for your business's future.

f) An employee timecard system: When you do choose to have employees, of course, you need a system for keeping track of the hours they work, so you can pay them. Handwritten sheets here cause all kinds of inaccuracies. So with my employees, I use an online app. Employees simply log in to punch in and punch out. It's much easier and keeps an accurate record of their entries.

As you learn more about on-site care, operating a clinic, and where your stressors are, you can change or add to these systems. For right now, however, thinking through these areas should eliminate some stress and get you off to a good start.

Remember that everything you need for your on-site clinic and for yourself when working should be stipulated in your contract. Good clients won't quibble over such costs—in fact, they'll be impressed by your thoroughness and organization. A good client wants you to have all the tools necessary to succeed. But they do need to know what those tools are, and that's on you. You are the professional here. It's up to you to lead your client when it comes to operating your on-site clinic.

YOU'RE IN BUSINESS

Thorough provisioning (or planning) in your work surroundings and supplies pays off in a multitude of seen and unseen ways. My business runs much differently than it did in the beginning thanks to my making that investment.

Today, I've given my office an entire room in my house—one with a door. I have a proper desk with an ergonomic office chair. When I'm working in my office, my laptop is connected to a regular-sized keyboard for more comfortable typing. I also connect the computer to a large monitor, so I can see and work on several documents at a time when needed. Not only can I leave my office "as is" at the end of a work session, I no longer worry about what's in the background when I have a Zoom call. (Nothing more humiliating than realizing there's a pile of unfolded laundry on the couch behind you as you talk with a client.) Making this investment in my space and equipment has improved my creativity, my productivity, and lowered my anxiety.

Just as important, having an efficient office and insisting on a well-equipped on-site space allows you to present yourself and your business as serious, dependable, and professional. Beyond making your job easier, you want every environment you work in-to emphasize to your clients and patients that you are a health care professional, someone who does things right, someone they can trust to take care of them. Proper space, proper equipment, and the right supplies go a long way in delivering that message and allowing you to do what you do best.

EXERCISE:
Create Your Spaces

Questions

1. Is there any part of having a home office that seems impossible to you right now? If so, what can you do to make it possible?
2. What piece of PT equipment do you consider a "must have"? How will this equipment be utilized in an on-site setting? Will it be a major or minor contribution to your services?
3. What opportunities come to mind when setting up your own clinic space? What will it feel like to move around that space and work with employees?

Activities

- Find and dedicate an appropriate space in your home for your office—and get it set up.
- Open a business bank account.
- Talk with your bank, CPA, and other small business owners, decide on accounting software, and then sign up for the software's free online class and take it.
- Check to be sure your current internet connection supports working from home—phone, computer, video meetings, other types of streaming.
- Create a master list with prices for the equipment you think you'll need on-site.
- Think through what systems you might want to put in place to relieve stress on your on-site operation.
- Buy yourself a pair of comfortable steel-toed shoes.

13

DAY ONE ON-SITE

So here you are—your business is up and running; you have a client and a signed contract with a plan in place. The next step is walking into your client's facility to open your first on-site clinic. Immediately on your arrival, there will be badge photos to be taken, security protocols to sign off on, safety procedures to become familiar with, a whirlwind of introductions, and a tour of the facility. Once those preliminaries are taken care of, you can head to your new office and treatment space and get them set up and ready to go. Expect everything to feel a bit clunky on this first day. New procedures and new surroundings always do.

Once your on-site office and clinic are in order, you'll want to head out to the floor to introduce yourself to the supervisors and other employees. Your brand-new safety shoes will probably feel a bit stiff, and your reflective vest might seem overly bright. But as you walk around and see people at work at their stations, you'll get the vibe of the place and begin to feel more comfortable.

Assume that most people you encounter won't understand what you do exactly or what having a physical therapist on-site means for them. So be prepared to explain yourself repeatedly. You might say something like, "I'm your on-site physical therapist. My clinic is right next to the break room. Your company is providing my services for you at no cost to you (or whatever the arrangement is). So whenever you have an ache or pain or any question about your health, just ask your supervisor for a few minutes of downtime to see the PT."

Slowly, employees will be curious and want to know more. Many, you'll find out, have never had access to physical therapy before, though they've needed it. Also, be ready for a few to ask you right away about an issue they're having. If practical, show them on the spot how you can help them to alleviate their pain with a stretch or better positioning; this is great for them and their coworkers to see physical therapy in action. If you're unable to solve their issue on the floor, invite them to come to the clinic when they can. Again, it's good for everyone to see how having an on-site PT works. The more familiar they can become with you and what you do, the more likely they are to reach out when they need to or when they have questions.

To that end, when I walked onto the floor at my first site, I went around with a stretch strap. As I introduced myself, I offered to show anyone who was interested how to use the strap for a nice anterior chest stretch, allowing them to experience for themselves how good PT can make them feel. So consider taking a stretch strap with you as you make your introductory rounds or maybe show them a self-massage technique, right there on the spot—anything to get employees associating your on-site PT clinic with taking care of pain and making them feel better.

By far the strangest part of the first day on-site for me was not having a full schedule of patients at my clinic door. It felt alarming not having a steady stream of work lined up, where I could see the expectations for the day and monitor my productivity. (All that seems kind of funny looking back on it, because when I worked at brick-and-mortar clinics, having people waiting for me was always such a huge source of stress.)

It didn't take me long to realize that the true measure of success for an on-site PT is to not have a line of patients waiting to be seen. We are there to prevent injuries, after all. As satisfying as it was and is for me to take care of a patient's pain, it's that much more rewarding to see that people don't get hurt in the first place because of an early intervention I provided.

As on-site PTs, we have creative control of our schedules. We can organize our days in ways that best achieve the client's goal of injury prevention and cost reductions. To that end, I always make sure I have regular and consistent times out in the work area for interaction with workers and ergonomic observations. I put systems in place to make the clinic itself more efficient. I also design and present programming to educate employees and their supervisors about how to protect their bodies on the job, as well as the warning signs of MSK injuries that they should have checked out by me at the clinic.

A FEW NEW BUSINESS DOs

You, of course, will find your own ways to fill your schedule and thus meet your goals and the needs of your patients and clients. Every company is different. Every contract is unique in its way. However, there are some universal principles that are good to know as you set out as an on-site PT, such as:

- DO create a to-do list for getting your business up and running properly. Use the chapters in this book to guide you. You'll find this list keeps you on track as you build toward getting that first client. If you should get a client before your business is totally put together (which does happen), this list becomes invaluable. Without it staring at you, reminding you that you are now an entrepreneur as well as an on-site PT, it's just too easy to get involved at the clinic and forget to tend to the business side of your business. As you complete each task, check it off the list. This will give you a visual that you are progressing, which in turn will give you the energy boost you need to keep going. (Personally, I love the feeling of checking things off a list.)

- As you move around your new on-site environment, DO keep a list of the various work areas. Note areas with the highest injuries or movement challenges. Those are the areas that need you, the areas where you can make a real difference for your patients and your client. Study them. Learn about the work done there and how it's done. Then, using your ergonomic assessment tools, design ways to monitor employee physical condition, decrease and prevent injury wherever possible.

- DO set up a regular meeting schedule with your client liaison (whomever you report to). Use this time to present issues you've noticed in the work areas, along with your suggestion for solutions. Remember to be a leader here. They've hired you as a professional to help them solve problems, so do that for them. At the beginning of your contract, make these meetings every two weeks or so. As trust builds and communication becomes easier between you and your liaison, these meetings can be reduced to monthly or even quarterly.

- DO keep up with your profession. Take the time to join professional organizations. Block some time to attend conferences (though not on days or during hours you are contracted to be on-site). Staying on top of the latest research, having relationships with your peers, and having other PTs to reach out to with questions benefits you, your client, and your patients. It's worthwhile.

- At the beginning of each year, DO be sure to schedule a vacation for yourself. You know and I know that if it doesn't get on your schedule, it will never happen. And it needs to happen.

- Remember, the only thing certain in business (and life) is change. So DO get in the mindset of going with the flow. You are going to make mistakes. Use them. See every challenge as another opportunity to learn and get better at what you do.

AND A FEW DON'Ts

- DON'T expect to be busy with patients on the first day or even the first month on a new site. Employees need time to figure out what you do, as well as when and how to use your services. It will take time for people to trust you.

- That said, DON'T sit in your office when you're not busy—not those first weeks, not ever. It's up to you to educate employees and supervisors about what their on-site PT clinic does and how you can help them. The first weeks are about YOU learning from the employees and how they work. Be seen. Be heard. Show yourself to be a team member.

- DON'T interrupt when an employee is explaining their job to you. They are the experts at their job, not you. Train yourself to be a good listener.

- The same goes for when a patient is telling you how they feel. DON'T interrupt. DON'T assume. One of the great luxuries of working on-site is that you have the necessary time with every patient. Take advantage of it. Get the whole story before you begin to formulate your clinical diagnosis and plan.

- DON'T email the client liaison incessantly with little things. You are the professional; figure it out and take care of it. Often employees and supervisors are better resources anyway. Usually, they can either help you immediately or they know exactly who to refer you to. If there are things you need to ask your liaison, keep a list and bring those items up at your regular meetings. If you can't wait, send one summary email with several questions.

FULL CIRCLE

At the end of your first day on-site, you'll pack up your safety gear and grab your keys. You'll leave the facility with no incomplete patient notes or clinic burdens hanging over your head. You'll head home knowing that you have made a difference for both your patients and your client.

For twenty years, being an on-site PT has brought me great satisfaction. I know I impact the lives of hardworking people for the better. Sometimes my impact comes in the form of relieving someone of a musculoskeletal issue that's been bothering them for years. Sometimes it's more systemic and changes a workflow or job function within the company—protecting dozens of workers now and many more in the future. Only by being an on-site PT would such opportunities ever have come my way.

As I said in Chapter 1, two decades ago, I was ready to quit the profession. Now, two decades on, I can't imagine anything I'd rather be doing. Sometimes I even have to take a deep breath because I can't believe what my career has grown into.

On-site PT saved my sanity and my health, to be sure. But it also has challenged me in ways I didn't know were available to physical therapists. Businesswise, I've built a solid practice. I employ other PTs and am able to provide them with a flexible schedule and above-standard pay. I mentor student physical therapists in effective treatment, as well as injury prevention and OSHA regulations. I solve complex problems for my clients that result in more efficient production, as well as substantial cost savings. And I still get to help individual workers feel better. At the end of my day, I lock the clinic door knowing that my efforts, skill, and talent matter. As an added benefit to me, at the end of each clinic day, my hands don't hurt, and I look forward to doing it all again.

Personally, I'm a much better human than I was before on-site PT came into my life. I spend a lot less time working, and yet, I'm financially better off and more financially stable. I've been able to return to the outdoor adventures I love with regularity. I have more time and more bandwidth for family and friends. All this has worked together to decrease my stress, which makes my brain and body work better both on the job and off. Most amazing, perhaps, I've become a more confident person in all aspects of my life.

Working on-site brought my career full circle—back to being a positive force—and allowed me to continue in a profession I felt and still feel called to.

NOW IT'S YOUR TURN

So now you have all the basics for building your own on-site physical therapy practice if you choose to. You have the tools, the business plan, and the inside scoop on what the job is really like and what you can expect. The only step left is committing to making it happen for you.

As I said in the opening chapter of this book, starting your own business can be intimidating. Especially when being an entrepreneur is not something you've ever considered before. Running a business will ask a lot of you—that is true. I hope what these pages have shown you, however, is that there's a prosperous return for that effort and the opportunity to come into your own in ways you never imagined. I hope you also know by now that you are more than capable of achieving and operating an on-site physical therapy practice if you want to.

The world and its workers need more on-site physical therapists. That's a fact. The field is only going to grow. Your future is up to you. You can do this.

EXERCISE:

Preparing for Your First Day

Questions

1. What are you looking forward to the most about your first day as an on-site PT?

2. What concerns do you have? Is there anything you can do now to relieve some of those concerns?

3. Is there anything on the "Do" list that feels overwhelming? Can you break it down and make it manageable?

4. Is there anything on the "Don't" list that feels hard? Again, can you break it down and make it manageable?

Activities

- Have a few standard questions to ask employees when you meet them. (Remember to listen to their answers.)

- Have a checklist of what you need to bring from your home office to your on-site clinic, so you don't forget anything.

- Take a moment to congratulate yourself on taking the leap to on-site PT.

14

AND ONE MORE THING . . .

I can't begin to count how often I say to patients, "And one more thing . . . let's try this." To me, that phrase and the frequency with which I say it are confirmations of the dynamic nature of what we do as physical therapists. Thinking on the fly. Observing and interpreting movement. Fine-tuning our in-clinic treatments, while simultaneously planning ways for the patient to have success on their own.

Therefore, it only seems appropriate to leave you with "one more thing" that I hope will drive home the breadth of the impact your work as on-site PT can have. Up until now, you've heard mostly from me about what on-site PT is and what it can do for your career and your life. Here, I want also to give you the opportunity to hear voices from the other side of the treatment table—words from those who contract with and oversee on-site care at their facilities, as well as from the patients who use our on-site PT services.

FROM MANAGEMENT . . .

James S.

James is the senior director of employee benefits at a large production facility. For more than two decades, he's been responsible for designing programs that impact employee health and managing the company's entire employee wellness experience. The two questions always at the top of his mind are: Is the program getting and keeping our employees healthy? Is the program cost-effective?

Here's what he has to say about on-site PT:

"If you just look at the amount paid for on-site PT versus the amount not spent (for community care), the financial ROI of on-site PT is nominal for a company. In this case, the VOI (value of investment) is the most important metric. When our on-site PT saves an employee from injury or a recordable, this can be estimated into a dollar value of money saved. And the employee perception of a caring employer, as well as low-cost and convenient services, is vital in the hyper-competitive labor market."

Dr. Philip Smaldone

Dr. Smaldone has been the medical director for a major international corporation for nineteen years. He finds on-site PT and IP services to be efficient, economical, and efficacious for the employees.

"The on-site services provide a convenient location near work for the employees, as well as greatly diminished cost to the employee when compared to off-site independent services. The on-site medical and PT services are an indication to our employees that their efforts for the company, along with their health and well-being, are valued. For me as a medical provider, the on-site services and the close working relationship with the therapists have allowed me to have confidence in their clinical outcomes. This allows me

to return employees back to work confidently and earlier than if at an off-site PT clinic. I wholeheartedly support the presence of PT and IP services on-site at the workplace."

Craig Snyder

Today, Craig Snyder, PE, CIH, CSP, is vice president of operations for an industry consultancy group. Before he moved up the corporate ladder, however, he was the safety manager at a large alcoholic beverage production/packaging facility, where I was the on-site PT. As safety manager, he was on the floor with me and witnessed the outcomes attained by having a physical therapist who understands the environment their patients work in. He was a staunch supporter of mine as I analyzed risks, designed task-specific programs, performed pre-employment testing, and as I cared for employees at their workstations.

Here are his impressions of on-site PT:

"If you want to build (company) culture, you must show employees you care. If management leads with that, it is a tremendous investment in the company and in the company's biggest resource, which is the employees. Providing care at the point of source through on-site clinics is smart and shows you care. Having a PT right there witnessing work-related exposures is priceless. You can't replicate that in a clinic environment. Having a PT providing support to occupational health clients on-site is the best and only way to do it super effectively."

Julie Chavez

Julie Chavez, PhD, CSP, has been in operational safety throughout her career. When I worked with her, she was a safety manager for a glass container facility. Her job was to ensure and document that the facility's safety programs worked to keep the employees safe and thus save the company money. She monitored safety culture, spending, and injury rates. In every company and environment that she's worked in, Julie has found the work of on-site PT's a real advantage in having a robust safety culture.

"In my career as a safety professional, preventing work-related illnesses and incidents has been the goal. And preventative measures—such as having on-site PTs— have been proven to be leading indicators in protecting em-ployees.

When I was environmental health and safety manager for a glass con-tainer manufacturer, I oversaw the safety of the forming team, who worked in extreme heat to produce 3.3 million bottles each day. Their work was so physically demanding, they were deemed industrial athletes. Having a PT dedicated to the site was imperative to ensuring the employees' health, as well as their safety. The PT monitored these employees for work hardening and heat acclimatization. The PT made ergonomic preventative interven-tions wherever needed.

As part of our risk assessment team, our on-site PT helped evaluate ergonomic and other safety issues throughout the plant. The findings were then used to help decide how to invest capital monies. They also complet-ed in-depth evaluations like the NIOSH lifting equation and the Snook Push Pull calculations, which provided quantitative measurements of risk. We then used that data to reduce injury through the redesign of machine guarding, box weight, and label positioning."

Cindy Trout

Cindy Trout works directly with workers' compensation claim managers as an occupational health case manager. In other words, she manages em-ployees who are absent from work due to illness or injury. Thus, she sees the many benefits to patients and employers of on-site care. These are her impressions:

"I can attest to the positive outcomes achieved with on-site PT. Having an on-site provider such as Chris and her team exceeds what the public sector can offer. They are an integral part of the (our) site's health and wellness team—everyone working together to restore the injured worker to their best level of function. Unlike outside health care providers, the on-site PT understands in a very real way the physical demands of the patient's job. Thus, their work with an injured patient naturally progresses into work conditioning and ensures a safe reentry into the workplace. With an on-site PT, quality of care, consistency of care, communication, and trust are unmatched."

Lucy Gilles Khouri

As senior wellness and health promotion manager for a large manufacturer, it's Lucy's job to incentivize workers to improve their health. She analyzes the effectiveness of where and how the company's wellness dollars are spent. In her view, on-site PT complements and supports her goals.

"Our on-site physical therapist has, time and again, proven to be the perfect partner for ensuring the well-being of our employees. Being out on the floor with us, our PT understands each employee's unique work situation and workspace setup. In addition, they provide effective integration with a medical plan of care—making it possible for injured employees to return to full work status more quickly and in a cost-effective way."

Ken Link

As a manager of a maintenance team, Ken works alongside his crew. Every day, he sees and experiences the benefit of the ergonomic work that having an on-site PT provides.

"As a manager, my employees, as well as myself, frequently are referred to our on-site PT for injury prevention assistance or treatment. This benefits the company through our increased productivity and decreased time away from the job. In addition, the employees are drawn into a wellness and self-care atmosphere. In any industry with maintenance and production, often there is heavy lifting to be done, along with awkward movements and strains that can cause injury. Being able to treat those issues without taking time away from work is a real benefit to the company and the employee. Also of note, with an aging workforce, I see the need for on-site PT as paramount."

WHAT PATIENTS SAY . . .

Tom Van De Bogart

An employee manager in finance—a desk job—Tom isn't the typical patient who utilizes the on-site clinic on the shop floor. However, his collegiate athletic career had caught up with him, as he was suffering from constant physical pain that was detracting from his work and slowing him down. When he noticed that the company's on-site physical therapy benefit was offered to all employees, he made an appointment. Not only did he find relief and better mobility through the treatment he received, but he became one of our clinic's biggest cheerleaders and a real advocate for on-site PT in general.

"I enthusiastically endorse employer-provided, on-site physical therapy—even for those of us who sit behind a desk. Competitive collegiate athletics unfortunately left me with some structural issues that resulted in two knee surgeries, a back injury, and hip replacements. Having the convenience of a talented PT like Chris in a preventative and rehab center at my worksite benefited both my employer and me. I can honestly say that

the treatment provided significantly delayed one surgery and prevented another. What a great employee investment that benefits both employees and the firm with preventative occupational issues!"

Kathy Motes

An IT director, Kathy found our on-site clinic when she was looking at her benefits package to see if her doctor-ordered PT would be covered. On-site PT made it easy for her to get the prescribed care without having to rearrange her schedule and take time off from work.

"I'd used off-site PT in the past. But with the on-site clinic, I found the ease of scheduling, the proximity, and most importantly, the connection I built with a consistent PT made for a quicker recovery. Chris and her team are highly regarded by employees from all areas of the business. At our company, they work with the doctors and personal trainers, who are also on-site, to provide a holistic approach to health care.

On-site physical therapy is a gift to the employee. It changes people's lives for the better. You get quicker attention to injuries, a better understanding of previous issues, and the building of trusted relationships."

Randy Sellinghausen

Randy's job is typical of the majority of patients you'll see on-site. A long-time maintenance worker, Randy suffered a fractured calcaneus after falling from a ladder (at home) in February 2020. After four months of being in a cast and numerous off-site doctor's appointments, he remained on restricted duty with no resolution to his injury. His leg remained swollen and purple. His HMO told him surgery wasn't available because of the pandemic—they suggested fusing his ankle, which he declined. Though his condition was not improving, his regular physician would not provide him with a prescription for physical therapy. As a last resort, he turned to his company's on-site medical clinic, which referred him to us at the on-site PT clinic.

This was his experience, in his own words:

"The on-site PT clinic was the best thing that could have happened to me. They helped to reduce the swelling in my leg, which had been getting worse since the injury. They taught me how to build muscle strength in my leg and how to balance. They showed me at-home exercises, which included bands, a rocker board, and a therapy ball. They also answered questions I had about my health and what recovery treatments would be like once I finally had surgery to fix the heel fracture. My on-site PT made me feel comfortable coming into the clinic. They listened to me and addressed each of my concerns without rushing through a session.

Another advantage of the on-site PT clinic is I didn't have to go back and forth from work to a doctor's office. My quality of life improved dramatically because I had an on-site clinic that I could turn to (and it may have saved my ankle.)

I always thought an on-site PT clinic was a standard service when you work for a corporation. But it is not the norm! How much productivity is lost because an employee has an injury and doesn't know how to get the treatments needed or where to turn for help? I now realize how lucky I am to have that option."

In addition to the direct care our on-site clinic could give Randy, we were also able to monitor his leg and ankle to ensure he'd be in the best condition when he finally was able to have the surgery he needed. It's cases like Randy's that make me grateful to be an on-site PT, where I can do my job thoroughly, with my only concern being the best outcomes possible for my patient.

As PTs, the care we give our patients is invaluable no matter the type of setting we practice in—helping them to move better, feel better, and providing them with the confidence needed to care for themselves moving forward. It's just that—as this entire book has emphasized—the structure of on-site PT care gives us the time, resources, and directive to provide that care in an optimal way. It allows us to use all our skill, all our talent, all our experience to do that "one more thing" to make our patients healthier, their workspaces safer, and our clients' businesses more productive.

It's not only valuable work but truly valued work. I feel that every day from both my clients and my patients. It's work I love. Here's to you loving it too.